Get Through
MRCGP – Clinical Skills Assessment

Bruno Rushforth MA(Cantab) MBChB MA
GP Specialty Registrar
West Riding GP Specialty Training Programme
Yorkshire Deanery

Val Wass BSc FRCGP FRCP MHPE PhD
Professor of Community Based Medical Education
Manchester Medical School
University of Manchester

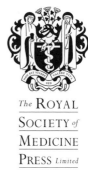

The ROYAL
SOCIETY of
MEDICINE
PRESS Limited

© 2008 Royal Society of Medicine Ltd

Reprinted 2008

Reprinted 2009

Published by the Royal Society of Medicine Press Ltd
1 Wimpole Street, London W1G 0AE, UK
Tel: +44 (0)20 7290 2921
Fax: +44 (0)20 7290 2929
E-mail: publishing@rsmpress.co.uk

British Library Cataloguing in Publication Data
A catalogue record for this book is available from the British Library

ISBN: 978-1-85315-736-3

Distribution in Europe and Rest of the World:
Marston Book Services Ltd
PO Box 269
Abingdon
Oxon OX14 4YN, UK
Tel: +44 (0)1235 465500
Fax: +44 (0)1235 465555
Email: direct.order@marston.co.uk

Distribution in USA and Canada:
Royal Society of Medicine Press Ltd
C/o BookMasters Inc
30 Amberwood Parkway
Ashland, OH 44805, USA
Tel: +1 800 247 6553/ +1 800 266 5564
Fax: +1 410 281 6883
Email: order@bookmasters.com

Distribution in Australia and New Zealand:
Elsevier Australia
30–52 Smidmore Street
Marrickville NSW 2204, Australia
Tel: +61 2 9517 8999
Fax: +61 2 9517 2249
Email: service@elsevier.com.au

Phototypeset by Phoenix Photosetting, Chatham, Kent
Printed in the UK by Bell & Bain Ltd, Glasgow

Get Through
MRCGP – Clinical Skills Assessment

		Dr	Pt	
	13	Is	N	
1	14	B	Is	←
2	15	N	B	
3	16	Is	N	
4	17	B	Is	←
5	18	N	B	

Contents

Foreword vii
Acknowledgements viii
Preparing for the Clinical Skills Assessment:
The 'why', 'what', 'when' and 'how' ix

Examination 1
Station 1 2
Station 2 12
Station 3 22
Station 4 32
Station 5 42
Station 6 52
Station 7 62
Station 8 72
Station 9 82
Station 10 92
Station 11 102
Station 12 110
Station 13 118

Examination 2
Station 1 128
Station 2 138
Station 3 148
Station 4 156
Station 5 164
Station 6 174
Station 7 182
Station 8 192
Station 9 200
Station 10 208
Station 11 218
Station 12 228
Station 13 238

Appendix 1 247
Appendix 2 249
Index 251

Foreword

From time to time books are published which every doctor studying the subject will have and refer to. I believe that this is such a volume. Although it is intended as a guide to the Royal College of General Practitioners Clinical Skills Assessment, it is also a wonderful guide to thinking holistically in a clinical setting and would be equally useful to medical students or any doctor working in a clinical setting which involves front-line care of patients.

The RCGP Clinical Skills Assessment tests a doctor's ability to assess and manage patients with common conditions; it also tests the candidate's ability to work effectively in a clinical setting. It is a test of performance rather than knowledge and so tests competence under a range of different pressures.

Each scenario in the book (there are 26) is a standalone revision of a common condition with up-to-date guidance of best practice management. It encourages the learner to think about different settings and how they would approach the presenting problem; readers are encouraged to consider what might lie behind the presenting problem and how they might use their interpersonal skills effectively. The book could be used for individual study or revision, but would be particularly useful as a basis for group study. It gives insight into the thought processes of our examiners and it encourages a holistic approach to study rather than a 'box-ticking' approach or rote learning. It approaches the Clinical Skills Assessment positively and encourages trainees to think about the domains which need to be assessed (and demonstrated) to assure the public of fitness for completion of training. It provides a helpful approach to the assessment, which would apply equally well to a busy surgery, such as moving to the next patient rather than dwelling on the previous consultation and making mental notes about revising knowledge when it is lacking.

I am certain that this will be a popular volume with trainees, trainers and programme directors.

Professor Jacky Hayden
Dean of Postgraduate Medical Studies
North Western Deanery and Manchester University
Principal in General Practice
Unsworth, Bury

Acknowledgements

We would like to thank the following individuals for kindly giving helpful feedback on earlier drafts: Amy Grundy, Rafik Taijbee, Wendy Brown, Nicola Cooper, Nat Wright, Jacki Barson, Linda Cusick and John Hamlin. We are particularly indebted to Amy Evans for constructive comments on all 26 scenarios. Thanks also to our models Rebecca Court and Sheena Ninan and to Windsor House Group Practice for allowing the use of their premises.

The editorial team at the Royal Society of Medicine Press has been supportive throughout and we are particularly grateful to Peter Richardson for his positive response to the initial proposal and to Sarah Burrows for accommodating our various requests.

We thank the individuals and publishing bodies that gave permission for us to reproduce extracts from their work. All are credited in the text.

Finally, we are very grateful to Arja Kajermo for her observant and witty illustrations.

Preparing for the Clinical Skills Assessment: The 'why', 'what', 'when' and 'how'

This chapter outlines the Clinical Skills Assessment (CSA) and offers a strategy for revision. We consider 'why' there needs to be a skills test, and discuss 'what' it involves and 'when' to apply to take it. Advice on 'how' to use this book to prepare for the CSA is then given.

Why a clinical skills assessment?

Formal examinations have come under increasing scrutiny now that it is acknowledged that assessment on performance in the workplace – i.e. what a doctor actually *does* – is the gold standard to aim for. The new MRCGP is no exception. There is now considerable emphasis on the e-portfolio of workplace-based assessment tasks that need to be completed throughout GP specialty training, supported by discussion and formative review with your trainer.

So why have an examination as well? The reasons are perhaps self-evident. We cannot yet be assured that assessments of performance are robust. The range of cases covered using the workplace-based tools will vary widely across different placements. The challenge of the tasks will differ as will the quality of judgements made by assessors. From the patient's perspective, the e-portfolio alone cannot assure a licensing body that the training curriculum has been covered. On the other hand, candidates in the past have not always felt their trainer has been fair. This can be difficult in the one-to-one supervision offered by general practice. Inevitably examinations must stay.

However, assessment is changing. There is an understanding that the methods selected to assess trainees must complement each other. The results need to be compared and integrated to ensure that a full and accurate perspective of the candidate's ability and level of performance is obtained. It is important to recognize this when studying for the CSA. Do not approach it in isolation as separate from the Applied Knowledge Test (AKT) or from your e-portfolio. The applied evidence-based knowledge tested in the AKT is essential to your performance in the CSA to demonstrate, for example, that you can use guidelines to reach appropriate management decisions. Formative assessments for the e-portfolio should be planned to inform your CSA preparation. Identical patient-centred, evidence-based, shared management structures underpin all components of the new MRCGP. Workplace-based assessment presents an ideal opportunity to get feedback on areas you are concerned about. Harness the thinking behind the new MRCGP to your advantage.

> View the CSA as part of an assessment package. Do not study for it in isolation.

Tips for preparation

1. Integrate preparation for the CSA with your e-portfolio.
2. Log your consultations. Identify gaps for revision against the curriculum.
3. Video your consultations from early on and discuss these regularly with your trainer.
4. Harness formative assessments with your trainer to develop your CSA skills.
5. Prepare carefully for case-based discussions using the suggested framework.
6. Use Mini CEX (Mini Clinical Evaluation Exercise) and DOPS (Direct Observation of Procedural Skills) to get feedback on all the listed clinical skills.
7. Reflect at the end of every surgery. Identify areas for improvement.
8. Make notes on consultations to use for revision and practise with colleagues.

What is the CSA?

The CSA assesses a *'demonstration'* of how you work when consulting in the surgery. You are invited to show the examiners how you would manage a range of simulated consultation scenarios in real life. If you prepare inadequately there is the danger of artificial rather than authentic performance.

You may have in the past revised for undergraduate Objective Structured Clinical Examinations (OSCEs) by memorizing check lists for the skills under test, grooming these on preparation courses or using books such as this one! Your rehearsed behaviours may not have related to your usual practice. Indeed, it has been argued that clinical tests can make 'monkeys of men', producing 'tick list' performances which score highly but are not at all reflective of actual practice. This can lead to faked behaviours and artificial performance. Preparation for this examination must be strategic and practice based to avoid this pitfall.

So why does the new MRCGP use an OSCE-type format? Do not be misled. This is a postgraduate examination and different. The CSA has been designed to test an integrated approach to the consultation based on real-life experiences. There is no check list to perform against or expectation of perfect performance. Your approach should mirror that of daily practice, i.e. patient-centred consultations resulting in appropriate shared management decisions. The assessment is designed to be as authentic as possible.

> Prepare in every day practice: aim for authentic not artificial performance.

The set up

The CSA consists of 13 standardized simulated consultations which test your ability to integrate consultation and clinical skills at an appropriate level of challenge. Each consultation is 10 min with a 3-min break in between. Piloting has confirmed that 12 stations are sufficient to ensure a reliable assessment of your performance. An additional station is inserted (anonymously) to pilot material for future use. The examination set up at least allows you to feel you are sitting in a surgery with the simulated patient (accompanied by the examiner) entering to consult with you. Focus on the patient and ignore the examiner.

> Observe your surroundings carefully on arrival: note the available equipment.

To embrace the full context of primary care the stations may include a telephone consultation and/or home visit. For example, you may be given a telephone in the break between patients, which rings at the start of the station, allowing you to consult with the simulated patient who is placed out of sight accompanied by the examiner. Alternatively, you may be taken, again in the 3-min break, into a room 'mocked-up' as the patient's house. At the end of this station you return to your consultation room.

Recommended equipment for your doctor's bag

You will be asked to bring a doctor's bag of basic equipment with you. Below is a summary of what this should include. Remember to take it with if you move stations for a home visit consultation.

- *British National Formulary (BNF)*
- Stethoscope
- Ophthalmoscope
- Auroscope
- Thermometer
- Patella hammer
- Sphygmomanometer (anaeroid or electronic)
- Peak flow meter and disposable mouth pieces
- Tape measure

The consultation process

There will be a set of basic notes for each consultation in a folder on the desk to read in the break between consultations.

> Read the patient information carefully, trying to formulate what is being tested.

A buzzer will sound to mark the beginning and end of each station. After the first buzzer, the patient will knock on the door or just enter, accompanied by an examiner. There are wall clocks in all rooms to help you judge the time. The consultation ends as soon as the second buzzer sounds – you cannot score any additional marks after this point. The simulated patient has been trained against a written script and the content can be covered in the allocated time. The tricky part is deciding whether a physical examination and/or clinical procedure (e.g. peak flow) are required. The examiner may guide you but do not rely on this. This is the only point in the process where they may interact. If you feel an intimate examination is indicated, you can suggest this although it should not be attempted unless a model is provided. If you say that you would like to examine the patient, then there are three possibilities:

- The patient may simply give you a card with the examination findings.
- The examiner may intervene and state – e.g. *"Assume the chest is clear"*.
- You will be required to carry out the appropriate examination and given any findings at the end.

This emphasizes the importance of the workplace-based assessments – e.g. the mini-CEX – in developing appropriate focused examinations through being observed and receiving feedback. Remember to gain consent for any examination and to explain the procedure to the patient.

Practise focused physical examinations using the workplace-based tools.

The marking system

The examiner silently makes an overall judgement in three performance domains of your ability to:

- **Domain 1: Interpersonal skills.** Integrate eliciting the patient's agenda and understanding of the problem with the specific information needed to make a diagnosis and shared decisions. Scenarios are designed to assess your ability to handle a range of patient emotions, ethical practice and demonstrate respect for equality and diversity.
- **Domain 2: Data gathering skills.** Elicit the appropriate information needed to make a clinical judgement on the patient's presenting problem, decide whether a physical examination is required and undertake this, supplementing it with other clinical procedures where appropriate.
- **Domain 3: Clinical management skills.** Recognize and manage common presenting complaints in general practice. These include undifferentiated problems, multiple complaints and issues which require a holistic approach to promote healthy living. You are expected to demonstrate a flexible, evidence-based and structured approach to decision-making with patients.

An overall mark for each station is then given: clear pass, marginal pass, marginal fail, or clear fail. Examiners are trained and have guidelines to standardize marking. However, they are making 'global' rather than 'check list' judgements. They are assessing your overall, integrated approach to the consultation, not ticking off a list of observed behaviours. The more experience you have gained in the surgery with your trainer, the more expert and natural your performance will be. Familiarity with a wide range of common presenting problems is essential. Only practice in the workplace will achieve this. We cannot emphasize enough the intentions of this marking system.

When should you take the CSA?

This is a matter for you and your trainer. We hope, however, that this book illustrates that it needs to be at a point when you have both a sound knowledge base and a fluent patient-centred consultation style. You must be able to apply guidelines using evidence-based practice and have sound diagnostic and consultation skills. Exploring the patient's agenda fully and formulating a shared patient plan must emerge naturally within your consultation. This requires experience and training using video feedback with your trainer and peers. You need to be well grounded in practice. The examination may feel like 'the surgery from hell' but you should have the experience to feel 'this is like being at work'. You should also have mastered the knowledge-base needed for general practice.

How does this book support you in preparing for the CSA?

This book offers two simulated tests of 13 stations, each with notes. We have designed a revision strategy to build a framework for your preparation. This aims to help you transfer skills from everyday practice into the simulated context of the examination. The notes after each scenario offer ideal approaches which cannot necessarily be covered fully in 10 min. We have aimed to paint a full picture. Remember the examiners are not looking for perfect consultations but a sound, integrated, well informed and patient-centred approach.

We strongly recommend you prepare with a group of peers. In addition to the cases in this book, try writing your own scenarios based on patients you see in surgery. Check the knowledge on which management decisions should be based and then offer them to colleagues for practice. The CSA is written from everyday examples and you will find you can do this just as well.

Step 1: Build a revision framework from the two test grids (see Appendices 1 and 2)

The scope of the curriculum is large. It is important you revisit this regularly on the RCGP website (www.rcgp.org.uk). We have designed grids to illustrate:

1. The skills being tested are devised from the marking criteria:

Category of skill

Gender mix	Age mix	Skills in diagnosis	Ongoing management skills	Clinical practical skills	Health promotion	Diversity and ethical issues	Dealing with patients' emotions

2. The contexts of common presentations which will be covered based on the curriculum.

Key for test grids: contexts covered based on the curriculum

Cardiovascular problems (CVD)
Digestive problems (GI)
ENT and facial problems (ENT)
Eye problems (Eye)
Metabolic problems (Endo)
Neurological problems (Neuro)
Respiratory problems (Resp)
Musculoskeletal system, including trauma (Rheum)
Skin problems (Derm)
Genetics in primary care (Gene)
Care of acutely ill people (Acute)
Care of children and young people (Paed)
Care of older adults (Geri)
Women's health (F)
Men's health (M)
Sexual health (Sex)
Care of people with cancer and palliative care (Pall)
Care of people with mental health problems (Psy)
Drug using adults (Drug use)
Promoting health and preventing disease (H Pro)
Care of people with learning disabilities (Learn dis)

We suggest you build a portfolio of consultations in your practice using these grids to identify the gaps in presentation and management you need to cover before sitting the CSA.

> Develop a grid to plot your own consultations, identify gaps for revision.

Step 2: Build a framework to formulate what the simulated consultation is testing

On first reading the station instructions to candidates, we encourage you to jot down, in the space provided, your initial thoughts on what is being tested before you read on. Commit yourself to doing this in anticipation of doing this in the CSA itself.

The full simulated patient scenario is then included to illustrate the importance of eliciting a comprehensive patient narrative to fully assess the purpose of the station. If you do not do this, key areas may be missed.

> Practise eliciting full patient narratives to ensure you don't miss hidden agendas.

Step 3: Work with the simulated patient

The simulated patient script has an additional purpose. Just as in real life a patient presents with a narrative (and we have encouraged you to record the ones you encounter in practice), so does the simulated patient. In the CSA these scenarios have been scripted to give the information needed to formulate diagnoses and management plans in the areas being tested. The simulated patient is not going to play 'cat and mouse' as patients sometimes unwittingly do. The information you require is in front of you waiting to be elicited. Ask open questions and the simulated patient can only respond as scripted. Responses to direct closed questions are also highlighted to illustrate the integration of data gathering into the interview. We use the scenario to highlight that it is crucial to listen sensitively in the initial phases of the consultation. Look for non-verbal cues as well. For example, in one station offered in this book, the patient has a packet of cigarettes in his breast pocket.

> The simulated patient has a script to deliver: use open questions initially to elicit this.

Step 4: Identify the full range of outcomes the examiner is looking for

After reading the patient's script, pause again and review what you now think the station is assessing. Again, there is space provided for you to make notes. We strongly recommend you do this. You should be able to formulate the issues the examiner is looking for under the headings: interpersonal skills, data gathering and clinical management. Then move on. The discussion section gives our expectations, which you can compare with your notes and discuss with colleagues. Remember you are aiming for sensible yet fluent coverage, not necessarily the ideal fully comprehensive scenario set out in the book.

> Aim in the 10 min to formulate a sensible fluent outcome: it will not be perfect.

Step 5: Your knowledge base

It is important to keep reviewing and updating your reading. It is a fallacy to view skills as distinct from knowledge. It is of paramount importance to patients that the information given and management decisions made are grounded in up-to-date evidence-based practice. We have outlined how each station links with the preparation you require for the AKT. The information is detailed. We acknowledge you cannot necessarily cover it all in 10 min. The aim is to illustrate how everyday practice can structure reading and revision for the CSA.

> Keep up to date with management guidelines: identify and 'plug' knowledge gaps.

Step 6: Write your own stations

We have aimed to offer a framework for doing this and ideas for further revision. Scenarios can be adapted to work with colleagues or alternative ones written.

> Use the book to develop your own scenarios for group revision.

Step 7: Finally

Why have so many stations if the marking schedule is a generic one? Herein lies a basic principle of assessment which has an important practical message. Doctors are not consistent in their practice. We are all good in some contexts and less good in others. Inevitably, however well prepared, you will perform better on some stations than others. It is crucial that you can handle this. If you feel you have done badly on a consultation, avoid using the 3-min break to reflect on this. Keep thinking forwards and focus immediately on the instructions for the next station where you may well perform brilliantly. We wish you well. Good luck.

> Think forwards in the CSA not backwards: some stations will be better than others.

Summary

Study the curriculum	Regularly review the curriculum. Keep up to date and evidence based. Make a grid to identify revision needs
Understand the skills	Develop well integrated clinical competencies. Do not work from checklists. Get feedback through direct observation or using video. Harness workplace based assessments
Practise the skills	The more experience the better; across a range of common presentations and a diversity of patients
Work with your peers	Revise together. Develop scenarios from everyday practice. Observe, role play, give feedback. It can be fun!
Use the CSA format	Use the breaks to think forwards, keep your eyes open, listen effectively and keep to the patient-centred, shared-management structure throughout
Remain confident	Develop the right mentality. You will undoubtedly 'flunk' some stations. Learn to move confidently onto the next

Examination 1

Stations 1–13

Examination 1: Station 1

Information given to candidates

> Wendy Morrison is a 30-year-old mother of two who works as an administrator and rarely sees her doctor. You note that her records show one episode of depression 6 years ago, which resolved without the need for medication or referral.
>
> She saw one of the other GPs in the practice last week complaining of feeling tired all the time. Physical examination was normal and urine dip-stick was negative.
>
> The results of her blood tests taken last week are:
>
> | | | | | | |
> |---|---|---|---|---|---|
> | Hb | 12.8 g/L | (12.0–15.0) | TSH | 2.12 mIU/L | (0.35–5.5) |
> | WCC | 7.5 × 10⁹/L | (4.0–11.0) | T4 | 18 pmol/L | (8–22) |
> | Platelets | 258 × 10⁹/L | (150–400) | | | |
> | | | | | | |
> | Na | 138 mmol/L | (135–145) | Glucose | 5.0 mmol/L | (4.0–6.0) |
> | K | 4.2 mmol/L | (3.5–5.0) | | | |
> | Urea | 4.2 mmol/L | (3.0–6.5) | | | |
> | Creatinine | 82 µmol/L | (60–125) | | | |

As the patient enters the consulting room she bursts into tears and says that she feels so low she "just can't go on".

- What do you think this station is testing?
- Make notes or discuss your thoughts with a colleague before you read on.

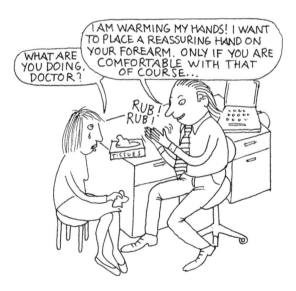

Plan your approach to this station:

Information given to simulated patient

Basic details – You are Wendy Morrison, a Caucasian 30-year-old female administrator.

Appearance and behaviour – You burst into tears as you enter the room. However, you soon recover your composure. You are well presented and maintain good eye contact during the consultation.

History

Freely divulged to doctor – You have been feeling low, slowed down and tired all the time for about 4 months. You are sleeping badly: finding it hard to get off to sleep and in the last month you have also been waking up at about 5 am and cannot get back to sleep, even though you feel exhausted.

Divulged to doctor if specifically asked – You were working 3 days a week but went full-time 6 months ago as money was tight and you and your husband are saving for a deposit on a house. Since then you have been finding it difficult to cope with the demands of running the home, looking after the children and working full-time. Your husband is sympathetic but is out at work himself much of the time. You had to give up your weekly get-together with friends as you just did not have the time to spare. You now find it hard to concentrate on things and your appetite is poor. You cannot seem to get any enjoyment out of the things you used to like, such as watching TV or reading. In the last week you have felt that you cannot go on like this, but you have never thought of hurting yourself in any way. You have never tried to hurt yourself in the past. You took today off work – your first day sick in 3 years – but told work that you had the flu. You came to see the doctor last week to say all this, but felt 'stupid' so did not mention your mood.

Ideas, concerns and expectations – You see yourself as a 'coper' and your family and friends describe you as a 'rock' in supporting them with all their problems. You feel 'weak' not being able to get well by yourself, and have put off coming to see the doctor. You have not told any family or friends that you are here today as you are embarrassed at seeking help for something that you think you should just 'snap out of'. However, you are frightened that your mood seems to be worse than when you were depressed 6 years ago. You are also worried at being labelled with a mental health problem and particularly do not want work to find out. You are hoping that the blood results will show some physical problem to explain your symptoms. If you need treatment for your low mood then you would prefer a 'natural' remedy, like St John's wort, rather than prescription tablets, but you want to talk to the doctor and find out more about this. You think 'counselling' with a 'stranger' would be a waste of time.

First words spoken to doctor – "I'm sorry doctor but I feel so low I just can't go on."

Past medical history – After the birth of your second child you felt low and tearful for several weeks and saw the doctor twice about this (on your mother's insistence). Things got better on their own and you put it down to the 'baby blues' and thought no more about it. You rarely see the doctor and have attended previously for pill checks and cervical smears.

Drug history – You are not allergic to any medication. You take the combined contraceptive pill – Microgynon 30.

Social history – You live with your husband and two sons – aged 6 and 8 – in a large rented flat. Your husband works as a self-employed shop-fitter. Your mother lives nearby and looks after the children after school. You drink the occasional glass of wine at home with meals. You have never smoked.

Family history – There is no history of mental health problems in your family.

- Having read the information given to the simulated patient, what do you now think this station is testing?
- Make notes or discuss your thoughts with a colleague before you turn the page.

Review your approach to this station:

Tested at this station:

1. Dealing with a distressed patient
2. Understanding a patient's illness experience
3. Taking a depression history
4. Self-harm risk assessment
5. Reaching a shared management plan
6. Appropriate follow-up and safety-netting

Domain 1 – Interpersonal skills

Dealing with a distressed patient

This patient is visibly upset. You need to spend the first part of the consultation quickly building an empathic, trusting relationship with her and exploring her distress:

- Allow the patient to speak uninterrupted and employ active listening skills, such as non-verbal communication, to demonstrate your interest and concern.
- Use silences to give the patient time to express her thoughts and feelings.
- Verbalize her distress – *"I can see that you're obviously upset"*.
- Paraphrase and summarize to demonstrate active listening and to help confirm your understanding.
- When a patient is upset, appropriate use of touch, e.g. on the arm, can act as a powerful show of support and empathy. However, this must be an authentic response to the situation rather than a forced move. Whether you choose to use it will depend on a number of factors, including the room set up, the rapport between yourself and the patient, your judgement on how it will be received, and whether you feel comfortable with such an act. If there is any doubt in your mind about the appropriateness of touch in any situation, then it is best not to use it.
- The new GP curriculum talks about finding a balance between emotional distance and proximity to the patient – in other words, be caring but stay objective and professional.

Understanding a patient's illness experience (overlap with Domain 2)

As medics, we are used to diagnostic categories, but these are the bare medical bones which you need to flesh out by building up a picture of the patient's own illness experience:

- Open questions are most appropriate to begin with to elicit the patient's story and to help you understand the patient's unique perspective.
- Explore the patient's ideas, concerns and expectations. How is her life affected by these problems? What are her own thoughts about what is making her feel like this? What most worries her about the current situation? Why did she not mention her mood last week when she saw your colleague? What does she want from seeing you today?

Domain 2 – Data gathering, examination and clinical assessment skills

Taking a depression history

Hopefully you will have obtained much relevant information from your initial open questions; however, you may need to follow these up with some more specific enquiries:

- Ask about mood, sleep, appetite, concentration, anhedonia (loss of capacity to experience pleasure), feelings of guilt, hopelessness and helplessness, and time off work.
- What support structures are in place to help her through this difficult time – friends, family, work?
- Does she have any anxiety symptoms? Depression and anxiety commonly co-exist.
- What has she tried to help? Does she feel anything has worked?
- What prescribed medication does she take? Remember that medication such as β-blockers can cause depression.
- You might also want to ask about alcohol and any illicit drug use as these can affect mood or be used as a coping strategy by patients.
- What happened during the previous episode of depression? How do things compare now to then?

Self-harm risk assessment

For any patient presenting with depression you must undertake a risk assessment for deliberate self-harm, which includes suicide:

- Be sensitive when asking about this subject – wait for an appropriate point in the consultation when you have built up rapport.
- *"How low have you felt at your worst?"* – is a useful opening question.
- Do not shy away from asking a direct question about whether the patient has ever thought about ending her life.
- Has she acted on any such thoughts? – e.g. made plans, written notes to loved ones, arranged her financial affairs.
- Any previous suicide attempts or other self-harm?
- You already know about her past medical history of depression, but have any close family members also had mental health problems?

Domain 3 – Clinical management skills

Reaching a shared management plan (overlap with Domain 1)

From reading the simulated patient information you will note that this patient has her own perspective on mental health problems and thoughts about treatment options. You should have elicited these during the consultation and should now attempt to incorporate her preferences when negotiating a shared management plan:

- Reassure her that the blood test results are normal. How does she feel about this?
- Ensure that you explain the diagnosis in simple, unambiguous terms. In this case it is *moderate depression*. What does she think of this?
- Explain how depression can affect things like sleep, appetite and concentration. Does she have any questions about this?
- Present various management options. What are her thoughts on these? Any worries about any of the options? They might include:
  - General advice on self-help measures such as exercise and sleep hygiene.
  - Seeking social support from family and friends. Is there any way she could start going again to the weekly get-together of friends?
  - St John's wort – the patient initially appears in favour of this treatment, but is she fully informed about this option? Does she understand that, although it can be effective in depression, it has the potential to interact with other drugs and it is difficult to know how much active treatment is present in certain preparations? Would you respect her wishes if, once fully informed, she still expressed a strong desire to self-medicate using St John's wort?
  - NICE guidelines (see Knowledge-base) list antidepressants as first-line treatment for moderate depression. If she decides to try antidepressants check for any drug allergies before prescribing. Advise her that she might initially feel more anxious or agitated and that it may take a few weeks before she notices any improvement. Warn her of common side effects such as gastrointestinal upset. Explain the potential withdrawal symptoms if she stops the tablets suddenly and that it is recommended to stay on the medication for at least 6 months after recovery.
  - 'Talking therapies' – e.g. cognitive behavioural therapy (CBT) with a psychologist. What does she think of this?
  - Time off work – advise her that she can self-certify for the first 7 days or, if she wants you to, you can write a sickness certificate for longer. If the latter, then you need to negotiate what to put down as the diagnosis. Is she happy for you to put 'depression' on the form?
- Would she like some written information such as a patient information leaflet on depression?
- Is the agreed plan mutually satisfactory – i.e. to patient and doctor?

Appropriate follow-up and safety-netting

Negotiating appropriate follow-up and what to do if things deteriorate is essential for those patients presenting with depression:

- Discuss with the patient that she should be seen again in 2 weeks, or earlier if she prefers.
- Ask if she would like the contact number of the local Crisis Mental Health Team. Let her know that she can call them anytime, day or night, if things get worse and she feels she needs immediate help.
- To make sure that follow-up arrangements have been fully understood, you could ask the patient to describe the plan back to you.

Knowledge-base – Management of depression

National Institute for Clinical Excellence (NICE) guidelines – Depression: management of depression in primary and secondary care. Clinical guidelines 23. December 2004 (amended 2007), www.nice.org.uk/CG023. Reproduced with permission.

	Who is responsible for care?	*What is the focus?*	*What do they do?*
Step 1	GP, practice nurse	Recognition	Assessment
Step 2	Primary care team, primary care mental health worker	Mild depression	Watchful waiting, guided self-help, computerized CBT, exercise, brief psychological intervention
Step 3 *The patient is currently at Step 3*	Primary care team, primary care mental health worker	Moderate or severe depression	Medication, psychological interventions, social support
Step 4	Mental health specialist, including crisis teams	Treatment recurrent, atypical and psychotic depression, and those at significant risk	Medication, complex psychological interventions, combined treatments
Step 5	Inpatient care, crisis teams	Risk to life, severe self-neglect	Medication, combined treatments, ECT

- Antidepressants are not recommended for the treatment of mild depression.
- Computerized CBT is an option for mild depression – e.g. Beating the Blues (www.ultrasis.com).

Take home messages

- How you relate to the patient – ideally showing respect and empathy at what is a difficult time for them – is more important than focusing your energies on an extensive checklist of questions.
- Risk assessment for deliberate self-harm must involve asking direct questions about thoughts of suicide.
- When negotiating a treatment plan, the key is to find out what the patient wants from coming to see the doctor.

Ideas for further revision

In primary care patients regularly present in distress or can become tearful during the consultation. After each such consultation, take a few moments to reflect on what you felt went well, and what you might have done differently, to help you better manage these emotionally-charged encounters.

Further reading

NHS National Library for Health Clinical Knowledge Summaries – Depression. www.cks.library.nhs.uk/clinical_knowledge.

NICE guidelines – Depression: management of depression in primary and secondary care. Clinical guidelines 23. December 2004 (amended 2007). www.nice.org.uk.

RCGP curriculum statement 13 – Care of people with mental health problems. www.rcgp.org.uk.

Information given to candidates

Steven Pinner is a 54-year-old electrician with asthma who failed to respond to two previous requests to see the practice nurse for an asthma review. His records state that he gave up smoking 20 years ago.

In the last 3 months he has had three repeat prescriptions for his salbutamol inhaler and four repeat prescriptions for his beclometasone inhaler.

He attended the local emergency department last week and the discharge sheet reads:

Patient: Steven Pinner

Attended St Benedict's emergency department complaining of 3-day history of:

- *Wheeze*
- *Worsening shortness of breath*
- *Chest tightness*

On arrival PEFR = 360 L/min (patient does not know best; predicted 590 L/min)
No features of acute severe asthma

ECG – sinus tachycardia
CXR – no abnormalities seen, awaiting formal reporting

Diagnosis – moderate asthma attack

Treated with O$_2$, nebulized salbutamol and oral steroids

PEFR post nebulizer = 520 L/min
Symptoms resolved, therefore discharged with 1-week course of prednisolone 30 mg OD

To see GP for follow-up

As the patient enters the consulting room you note that he has a packet of cigarettes in his shirt pocket.

- What do you think this station is testing?
- Make notes or discuss your thoughts with a colleague before you read on.

Plan your approach to this station:

Information given to simulated patient

Basic details – You are Steven Pinner, a Caucasian 54-year-old male electrician.

Appearance and behaviour – You have a packet of cigarettes in your breast shirt pocket.

History

Freely divulged to doctor – Your breathing has been getting worse over the last 3 months. Your partner said that she could hear you wheezing when you arrived back from a walk to the corner shop. You know that this is probably because you have started smoking again. You went to the emergency department 5 days ago as you were finding it difficult to get your breath when you woke up one morning. They gave you oxygen and some medication through a mask. Your symptoms improved so you were sent home with a supply of steroid tablets.

Divulged to doctor if specifically asked – You did not make a conscious decision to start smoking again but just 'fell into it' when you moved in with your partner 3 months ago and this 'set off' your asthma. You were waking with a cough two or three times a night and you felt short of breath and wheezy climbing a flight of stairs. You have not coughed up any blood or phlegm, but your chest felt tight when the breathing was bad. You felt much better after having the treatment in hospital. Your breathing has been good since you were discharged and you went back to work 2 days after attending the hospital without any problems. You have cut down to about 10 cigarettes a day since leaving hospital. You meant to respond to the asthma nurse review letters but find it difficult to get time off work to attend appointments. You cannot remember the last time you had your peak flow checked or what it was. Twenty years ago a family friend who smoked heavily died of lung cancer and when you heard this you decided to quit smoking, which you did the same day without any help.

Ideas, concerns and expectations – You were frightened by the asthma attack last week as nothing like that has ever happened before. You were taking at night the steroid tablets given to you by the hospital but you felt they disturbed your sleep so you stopped taking these after 3 days (you had been told to take six tablets each day for a week). You want to stop smoking but feel you need help with this, especially as your partner smokes but does not want to stop, and this is causing arguments at home. Since you started smoking again you have been thinking about the family friend who died of lung cancer and how you might go the same way if you don't quit. You did try and make an appointment to see the practice nurse who runs the smoking cessation clinic but you could not get through on the telephone. You are hoping that the doctor today will be able to give you some help with stopping smoking; you have heard about nicotine patches and gum.

First words spoken to doctor – "The hospital said that I should come and see you about what happened."

Past medical history – You had 'keyhole' surgery on your left knee 12 years ago to remove damaged cartilage after you slipped and fell. You have had antibiotics from the GP for chest infections on a couple of occasions over the last 5 years. Otherwise you are normally fit and well.

Drug history – You have two inhalers: a blue salbutamol inhaler and a brown beclometasone inhaler. You rarely used either of them until 3 months ago. Since then you had been using each of them up to eight times a day, but you don't really understand the difference between the two. You have used the blue and brown inhalers only twice each since leaving hospital. You are not allergic to any medication.

Social history – You are divorced from the mother of your two sons, and had been living on your own for 5 years until you moved into your female partner's terraced house 3 months ago. You have been in the same job for over 10 years. You drink five or six pints of beer over the weekend at the pub with friends.

Family history – You have two adult sons, neither has asthma but one has eczema.

Review your approach to this station:

Tested at this station:

1. Understanding a patient's illness experience
2. Data gathering and examination
3. Chronic disease management
4. Smoking cessation advice
5. Reaching a shared management plan

Domain I – Interpersonal skills

Understanding a patient's illness experience

The patient has had a recent scare with the deterioration of his breathing and asthma attack. How you elicit the patient's story and address his fears and concerns are key skills:

- Start with open questions to allow his story to unfold.
- How does he feel after the hospital visit? What was it like being rushed to hospital? Has it affected how he views his asthma?
- What are his thoughts about having started smoking again? Does he have any worries about this? – e.g. concerns about lung cancer.
- Have recent events impacted on his work or home life? – e.g. arguing with his partner.
- What does the patient want from the appointment today – what is his agenda?
- Are there any specific questions he wants answered? – e.g. concerns about steroid use.

Domain 2 – Data gathering, examination and clinical assessment skills

Data gathering and examination

Although the consultation needs to be patient-centred, you will have your own agenda too, with specific questions about the history and examination to cover before you feel happy to come to a shared management plan:

- Elicit the history building up to his attendance at hospital – How was he sleeping? Was he wheezy or short of breath? Any chest pain? Was he bringing up phlegm?
- Explore why his asthma has deteriorated over the last few months. Find out about triggers – e.g. smoking, recent chest infections, moving house, new job, pets, new drugs or over-the-counter medications (aspirin, non-steroidal anti-inflammatory drugs [NSAIDs] and β-blockers can all make asthma worse).
- A good screening question if you suspect that his symptoms are related to his occupation is – "*Do your symptoms improve when you are not at work or on holiday?*"
- Any red flag signs – e.g. weight loss or haemoptysis?
- Given the patient's age, history of smoking and chest tightness, it may be worth asking some cardiac screening questions.

- How have things been since leaving hospital? Has he been using his inhalers and has he taken the tablets prescribed?
- Checking his peak flow could give both you and the patient further reassurance and help establish a baseline reading.
- If his symptoms have resolved and you are happy with his peak flow, then further examination is probably not required.

Domain 3 – Clinical management skills

Chronic disease management

This station will test key clinical skills in working in partnership with patients to improve their chronic disease management:

- Assess the patient's understanding of his condition.
- What are his thoughts about managing his condition?
- What is important to him about his asthma? – e.g. symptom management.
- Does he understand how his inhalers work? What is his inhaler technique like?
- Does he ever use a peak flow meter to monitor his asthma? Can he use one correctly?
- Are there any barriers to him coming to regular asthma review appointments?
- Does he understand what to do if his symptoms worsen?
- You could motivate the patient in self-management by empowering him to adjust his medication as appropriate.
- Providing details of self-help support groups and national organizations would allow him to access peer support and advice – e.g. Asthma UK (www.asthma.org.uk).
- You could offer to provide written material to reiterate the points above – e.g. a personalized, written asthma action plan – or use diagrams or models to aid explanations. Check what is in front of you on the desk at this station.

Smoking cessation advice

Smoking cessation advice is a proven cost-effective intervention in primary care, and is all the more important for those with chronic respiratory conditions:

- Where is the patient on the 'cycle of change'? In this case he has relapsed, but is contemplating trying to stop again.
- Be extremely positive about any comments he makes about wanting to quit.
- Explore his reasons for stopping smoking previously and emphasize the benefits for his health – use the example of the recent asthma attack to reinforce this point.
- Did he find anything useful last time that helped him stop smoking? His concerns about lung cancer acted as a powerful motivator previously.

- Does he know about the help available now? – e.g. nicotine replacement therapy and external smoking cessation programmes or nurse-run practice smoking cessation clinics.
- You could reassure him that many people relapse, but can still quit again and stay a non-smoker.

Reaching a shared management plan (overlap with Domain I)

The key here is to come to an acceptable management plan that suits this patient's particular life circumstances:

- Try and incorporate the patient's health beliefs into the management plan – e.g. *"Yes, you're right that smoking is making your asthma worse – trying to stop would be the best thing you could do for your health."*
- Present options which are both realistic and fit with the patient's agenda and priorities. Discussing his thoughts about the way forward is essential. Options might include:
  - Referral to the smoking cessation clinic.
  - Agreeing to review whether to step up or step down his medication after he has attempted to stop smoking (see Knowledge-base).
  - Prescribing a peak flow meter with a diary card to allow self-monitoring.
  - Reassurance that nothing suggests a sinister cause of his recent deterioration – e.g. lung cancer. You could offer to let him know when you receive the results of the formal chest X-ray report.
  - Reassurance that steroid tablets for short term use are safe but best taken in the morning to avoid insomnia.
  - Referral to the nurse for spirometry to assess whether there is any component of chronic obstructive pulmonary disease (COPD) to his condition.
  - Providing information on what to do if his symptoms worsen.
  - Regular follow-up at the nurse-led asthma clinic.

Knowledge-base – Management of asthma

BTS & SIGN British Guideline on the Management of Asthma (adults). Updated November 2005. www.brit-thoracic.org.uk. Reproduced with permission.

Step 1	Step 2	Step 3	Step 4	Step 5
Inhaled β_2-agonist as required, e.g. salbutamol, terbutaline	*Patient is currently at Step 2 of the guidelines* Add inhaled corticosteroid, e.g. beclometasone 200–800 µg/day	Add inhaled long-acting β_2-agonist (LABA), e.g. salmeterol **Good response** to LABA, continue LABA **Partial response** to LABA, increase steroid dose to 800 µg/day* **No response** to LABA, stop LABA and increase steroid dose to 800 µg/day.* If control still inadequate, trial other therapies, e.g. leukotriene receptor antagonist or theophylline	Consider trials of: Increasing inhaled steroid dose up to 2000 µg/day* Addition of fourth drug, e.g. leukotriene receptor antagonist, theophylline, β_2-agonist tablet	Daily steroid tablet in lowest dose for adequate control Maintain high dose inhaled steroid at 2000 µg/day* Consider other treatments to minimize use of steroid tablets Refer patient for specialist care

*Beclometasone dose or equivalent.

- You should titrate inhaled steroids to the lowest dose for effective control of symptoms.
- LABA inhalers should not be used on their own, but in combination with inhaled corticosteroids.
- Consider a trial of stepping down treatment if symptoms are well controlled.

Take home messages

- It is important to discover and address the patient's health beliefs and behaviours.
- In chronic health conditions such as asthma, patient education, motivation and encouraging self-management are key.
- Safety-netting and appropriate follow-up are essential when dealing with potentially life-threatening conditions.

Ideas for further revision

In the CSA there will be a balance of acute and chronic presentations. This station is an example of an acute exacerbation of a chronic condition. Chronic disease management is a key skill expected of GPs, so you should ensure that you feel confident with the management of common chronic conditions seen in primary care, such as diabetes, COPD, asthma and osteoarthritis.

Further reading

Asthma UK. 'Be in Control' – free pack containing personal asthma action plan for patients. www.asthma.org.uk.

RCGP curriculum statement 15.8 – Clinical Management: Respiratory problems. www.rcgp.org.uk.

The British Thoracic Society (BTS) & Scottish Intercollegiate Guidelines Network (SIGN) British Guideline on the Management of Asthma (adults). Updated November 2005. www.brit-thoracic.org.uk.

Information given to candidates

Mrs Evans is a 44-year-old mother of three who has asked to see the doctor to talk about her youngest son Steven, aged 11.

She is attending without her son today.

Steven's records show:

Normal birth and development.

PMH – asthma. On beclometasone and salbutamol inhalers.
Sees the asthma nurse regularly – no concerns, good control of asthma.

Other attendances at the GP have been for minor self-limiting illnesses.

BMI noted to be at 91st centile on last attendance.

As Mrs Evans enters the room she says, "I'm sorry to bother you doctor but I'm worried about Steven's weight."

- What do you think this station is testing?
- Make notes or discuss your thoughts with a colleague before you read on.

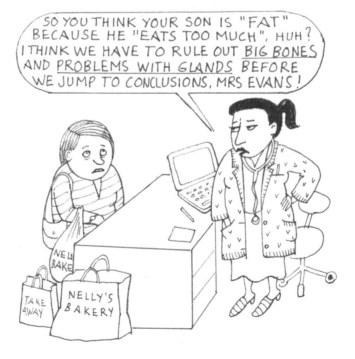

Plan your approach to this station:

Information given to simulated mother

Basic details – You are Janet Evans, a Caucasian 44-year-old mother of three who works part-time in the local baker's.

Appearance and behaviour – You are overweight, well presented and a little anxious.

History

Freely divulged to doctor – You have found out through a friend, whose daughter goes to the same school as your youngest son Steven, that he is being teased at school about his weight, with other children calling him 'fatty'. Steven has always been a 'heavy' boy but has put on weight over the last year and now seems to weigh more than his 13-year-old brother (although you do not know his exact weight as Steven refuses to go on the scales – he can be a bit sensitive about this). You have tried to get him to play outside more, but his brothers also like to stay in and watch television or play on the computer, and he has always looked up to, and followed, them. He has even stopped going out with his grandad on the long walks they used to do together.

Divulged to doctor if specifically asked – The family rarely sits down in the evenings to eat together at the kitchen table. Instead the children and your husband eat in front of the television in the front room. You usually eat in the kitchen to get some peace and quiet. In the past you have tried to buy more healthy foods but the children complain that they do not like them. Despite you and your husband working, money is tight so you often shop at the local budget store, which does not sell fresh fruit or vegetables. You tend to buy the more convenient pre-prepared meals as there is often no time to do a 'proper' meal. Steven is doing fine academically and has always come above average in his marks at school. Steven has a small group of friends at school, but has seen less of them recently outside school. Steven used to play table tennis regularly at the local youth centre but gradually stopped going last year. Steven has not complained of any aches or pains, and you have not noticed any problems with his mood. He has not wet the bed since he was a toddler. Steven's asthma is well controlled by his inhalers and he regularly attends the asthma nurse clinic at the GP surgery. Apart from his asthma and weight, you have no other health concerns regarding Steven. Lunch at school is provided by the canteen, and you give Steven money for this, although you suspect that he goes to the chip shop instead. Most members of the family are 'heavy', but you only think of Steven as having a problem with his weight. You did not bring Steven today as you first just wanted to discuss things on your own with the doctor.

Ideas, concerns and expectations – You believe that Steven's problems are probably due to eating too much and not doing enough exercise, but you are also worried that his steroid inhaler may be increasing his appetite. You feel a little guilty that if you gave him healthier foods then he would probably not be overweight. You think that taking him to Weight Watchers might be a way forward, but want to know what the doctor thinks about this – is he too young? You are hoping that the doctor will be able to allay your fears about any serious cause for the weight gain, and to suggest some ways to tackle it.

First words spoken to doctor – "I'm sorry to bother you doctor but I'm worried about Steven's weight."

Past medical history – You have been on antidepressants for 8 months, but your mood has been good for some time now and you are planning to see the doctor about coming off the medication.

Drug history – You take fluoxetine 20 mg once a day for depression.

Social history – You live with your husband and three children in a council house. You and your husband drink the occasional glass of wine or beer. Neither of you smokes. You work 4 days a week from 10 am to 4 pm at the local baker's and often bring back unsold cakes from work. Your husband works as a roofer. You have a strong marriage. You do all the cooking for the family. Your three sons – Michael 15, James 13 and Steven 11 – get on well together. You drive them the two miles to and from school every day. You rarely do physical activities – such as swimming or going on walks – as a family.

Family history – There are no major health problems in the immediate family.

- Having read the information given to the simulated mother, what do you now think this station is testing?
- Make notes or discuss your thoughts with a colleague before you turn the page.

Review your approach to this station:

Tested at this station:

1. Dealing with a third party
2. History taking skills
3. Health promotion and lifestyle advice
4. Reaching a shared management plan

Domain 1 – Interpersonal skills

Dealing with a third party

There are always difficulties in conducting a consultation about a patient who is not actually present. In fact, your primary role is often to address the third party's concerns – usually a relative or spouse – rather than dealing with the absent person's 'problem'. Particular issues to consider in this case include:

- Mrs Evans is worried about her son's weight and that he is being called names at school, but you do not know to what extent Steven is particularly bothered by this. You could explore this with her.
- Mrs Evans appears anxious. As you discuss her concerns regarding her son you need to address, and if possible allay, her anxieties.
- Do you detect any feelings of personal responsibility – or guilt – for Steven's weight gain?
- You could positively reinforce her attendance today by saying how she's made the first step to try and help Steven.

Domain 2 – Data gathering, examination and clinical assessment skills

History taking skills

You need to try and obtain as comprehensive a history as you can from Steven's mother about his weight gain:

- When did she first notice a problem with his weight?
- How much physical exercise does Steven do? Any sports? Does the family ever do activities together such as swimming or walks?
- What sort of food does Steven eat? Does he eat foods with high sugar and fat content? Does he eat foods rich in salt? How often does he eat fresh fruit and vegetables?
- Where does he eat meals? Do you ever find evidence of Steven eating secretively?
- How is he getting on at school? Has he mentioned the name calling? Any concerns raised by his teachers? Does he have any educational or learning difficulties?
- Does Mrs Evans have any worries about his mood?
- What are her beliefs about eating, activity and weight?
- What is the whole family's lifestyle like? Is Steven's eating behaviour any different from his siblings?
- What does Mrs Evans' husband think about Steven's weight? What are his views about the family's lifestyle? What are the other children's views?

- Although Steven is not actually present, have you managed to exclude any obvious serious pathology from taking a history from his mother? – e.g. you could ask about symptoms such as:
  - Headache and visual disturbance
  - Thirst and polyuria
  - Constipation and fatigue
  - Early-onset puberty
  - Striae and central obesity
  - Family history of endocrine disorders.

Domain 3 – Clinical management skills

Health promotion and lifestyle advice

It is important that parents take some responsibility for lifestyle factors in the home, such as diet and eating behaviour, if change is to happen. Points to discuss with Mrs Evans could include:

- How willing is the family to change lifestyle? Without a positive attitude to change it is unlikely that any modifications will be sustainable.
- Multicomponent interventions are the most effective at tackling obesity – in other words, it is important to address a whole range of unhealthy behaviours, rather than just focus on, say, diet.
- Increased physical activity – aim for a total of 60 min of moderate activity each day. Are there any sports that Steven enjoys but has not done for a while? How might he be encouraged to take these up again?
- Reduce physical inactivity – aim for a limit on the time spent playing computer games or watching TV each day.
- Improve eating behaviour – such as eating together as a family at the table.
- Healthy eating – base meals on starchy foods such as potatoes, rice, pasta and bread and aim for five portions of fruit or vegetables each day. Look to cut down on high fat and high sugar foods and drinks.
- Behaviour change strategies – such as goal setting, praise and rewards, and self-monitoring can all help. Has Mrs Evans tried any of these with Steven?
- What are the barriers to Mrs Evans and her family adopting a healthier lifestyle? – e.g. cost, availability of facilities – such as a local leisure centre – and other family members' attitudes. How might these be overcome?
- Adopting a healthier lifestyle could help the whole family in the long term by reducing the risks of heart problems, arthritis and diabetes.

Reaching a shared management plan (overlap with Domain I)

For any plan to be effective you need to make sure that you have taken into account the patient's needs and preferences. In this case you need to think about the whole family as behavioural change is unlikely to be effective unless it is a joint endeavour. Options you could suggest to Mrs Evans as a way forward include:

- Asking Steven to come in to see you for a chat, to allow you to conduct a proper assessment, including taking baseline weight and height readings. You need to feel happy that there is no other pathology causing his weight gain.
- Speaking to Steven on his own could reveal his own thoughts and feelings about his weight. These need to be incorporated into any management strategy.
- Lifestyle changes for Steven and the whole family in small, manageable and realistic steps might include:
  - Walking to school rather than taking the car. Does Mrs Evans think this is feasible?
  - Organizing regular family activities such as going swimming or for walks with grandad. Are there any activities the whole family enjoys that involve some physical exertion?
  - Agreeing a limited time spent on the computer each day. Would this be enforceable?
  - Giving Steven and his brothers packed lunches rather than money which can be spent on unhealthy foods. How would the children react?
  - The family agreeing to eat the evening meal together at the kitchen table. What would the family think about this?
  - Mrs Evans not bringing home unsold cakes from her work at the baker's.
- Referral to a dietician for further advice and support – such as with meal planning and shopping.
- Using self-help or commercial weight management programmes should only be considered if they are based on a balanced diet, encourage exercise and do not promise excessive weight loss. Mrs Evans may wish to try simple strategies to help improve Steven's lifestyle first.

Knowledge-base – Assessment and classification of overweight/obesity

National Institute for Health and Clinical Excellence (NICE) clinical guidelines 43: Obesity – Guidance on the prevention, identification, assessment and management of overweight and obesity in adults and children (Quick Reference Guide 2). December 2006. www.nice.org.uk/CG043. Reproduced with permission.

Determine degree of overweight or obesity
- Use clinical judgement to decide when to measure weight and height
- Use BMI; relate to UK 1990 BMI charts to give age- and gender-specific information
- Do not use waist circumference routinely; however, it can give information on risk of long term health problems
- Discuss with the child and family

↓

Consider intervention or assessment
- Consider tailored clinical intervention if BMI at 91st centile or above
- Consider assessing for co-morbidities if BMI at 98th centile or above

↓

Assess lifestyle, co-morbidities and willingness to change, including:
- Presenting symptoms and underlying causes of overweight or obesity
- Willingness to change
- Risk factors and co-morbidities – such as hypertension, hyperinsulinaemia, dyslipidaemia, type 2 diabetes, psychosocial dysfunction, exacerbation of asthma
- Psychosocial distress – low self-esteem, bullying
- Family history of overweight, obesity and co-morbidities
- Lifestyle – diet and physical activity
- Environment, social and family factors
- Growth and pubertal status

↓

Management
Offer multicomponent interventions to encourage:
- Increased physical activity
- Improved eating behaviour
- Healthy eating

Consider referral to a specialist if the child has:
- Significant co-morbidity, or
- Complex needs such as learning or educational difficulties

- Surgery or appetite suppressant medication are not recommended for children.

> **Take home messages**
> - Taking a history from a third party can be problematical – encourage the patient to attend for proper assessment.
> - Being positive and encouraging change in the whole family is important when trying to help support healthy lifestyle choices for patients.
> - Interventions for obesity are more likely to be effective if they are multicomponent – i.e. address diet, eating behaviour and physical activity together.

Ideas for further revision

The CSA, at least initially, is unlikely to use child-simulated patients. In order to cover paediatric cases you will therefore be presented with third parties – e.g. a worried parent – attending on their own or telephoning for advice. Think about how these scenarios might be set up – e.g. a telephone consultation about a child at home with diarrhoea or parental concerns about self-harm, drug misuse or an eating disorder in their adolescent son/daughter. Next, identify what you would need to know and do, in order to score highly at such a station.

Further reading

National Heart Forum and Faculty of Public Health – Lightening the load: tackling overweight and obesity 2006. www.fphm.org.uk/policy_communication/publications/toolkits/obesity/default.asp.

NICE clinical guidelines 43: Obesity – Guidance on the prevention, identification, assessment and management of overweight and obesity in adults and children. December 2006. www.nice.org.uk/CG043.

Information given to candidates

> Julie Matcham is a 23-year-old woman who works for a public relations company.
>
> Her notes show that she has been seen twice over the last year with 'mild acne' and has been treated with:
>
> - Topical benzoyl peroxide 5% BD prescribed 10 months ago
> - Oral antibiotics – doxycycline 100 mg OD – commenced 10 days ago
>
> Her past medical history includes irritable bowel syndrome.
>
> For the purpose of the exam, assume that today the patient has mild acne on her face only.

As the patient enters the room she says, "I was hoping that you could send me to see a skin specialist."

- What do you think this station is testing?
- Make notes or discuss your thoughts with a colleague before you read on.

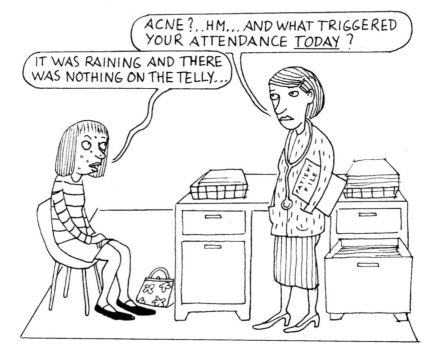

Plan your approach to this station:

Information given to simulated patient

Basic details – You are Julie Matcham, a Caucasian 23-year-old recent graduate who works in public relations.

Appearance and behaviour – You appear confident and articulate. You have mild acne on your face only.

History
Freely divulged to doctor – You want to see a skin specialist so you can be prescribed the drug Roaccutane, as you have tried creams and antibiotic tablets for your acne but you think your acne is still bad. From looking on the internet you know that your GP cannot prescribe Roaccutane and that you have to be referred to a specialist first.

Divulged to doctor if specifically asked – You had problems with acne as a teenager but only ever used over-the-counter creams. Things flared up about a year ago, soon after you left university and started working, but the acne got better after a month of using the cream prescribed by your GP, so you stopped using it. Ten days ago you saw the GP again as you thought the acne had returned and you were prescribed antibiotic tablets. You know that you are meant to come back in 6–8 weeks for a review, but you feel that things have got worse since you were last seen. When you were back at your parents' home last week you tried using some of your brother's eczema cream, but this just seemed to aggravate your skin. You are otherwise well. Your mood is OK, although you feel less confident at work, due to your skin. Your periods are regular and you have not noticed any excessive facial hair growth. To your knowledge, no family members have polycystic ovary syndrome. You split up with your boyfriend last week and are still upset about this. You think that your boyfriend may have left you because of your acne, although he always said that he thought your skin was fine.

Ideas, concerns and expectations – A friend mentioned Roaccutane as a possible treatment for acne – although she had only read about it in a magazine. You are worried about having scars if the acne is not treated properly. You think that your acne may have been the reason that you were switched from managing one client to a less high profile one at work, although your boss explained that the move was due to sickness cover. You are very keen to be referred to a specialist to obtain the Roaccutane. However, if the doctor offers you other options for managing your acne and comes across as understanding and competent, then you will consider these.

First words spoken to doctor – "I was hoping that you could send me to see a skin specialist."

Past medical history – You suffer from irritable bowel syndrome – a feeling of having a bloated abdomen, lower abdominal pain relieved by opening your bowels, and intermittent diarrhoea and constipation – although these symptoms have not bothered you much recently.

Drug history – You have been taking antibiotic tablets – doxycycline 100 mg, one tablet once a day – for 10 days. For several years you have been taking the combined oral contraceptive pill, Microgynon 30. You do not remember the doctor who prescribed the antibiotics asking whether you took the pill or informing you that you should take extra contraceptive precautions while you are taking the antibiotics. You also take vitamin supplements and occasionally paracetamol for headaches. You are not allergic to any medication.

Social history – You have been working as a new graduate recruit in a public relations firm for about a year. You were living with your boyfriend until recently, when he ended the relationship, and you now share a rented flat with two other friends. You have not been going out socializing as much as usual recently as you feel more self-conscious about your skin. You have been wearing more make-up recently to try and hide your acne.

Family history – Your brother has eczema. There is no family history of serious health problems.

- Having read the information given to the simulated patient, what do you now think this station is testing?
- Make notes or discuss your thoughts with a colleague before you turn the page.

Review your approach to this station:

Tested at this station:

1. Understanding the patient's illness experience
2. Identifying a hidden agenda
3. Data gathering
4. Dealing with a referral request
5. Reaching a shared management plan

Domain 1 – Interpersonal skills

Understanding the patient's illness experience

Some dermatological presentations in primary care can appear trivial to doctors, but the GP curriculum stresses the importance of recognizing the social and psychological impact of skin problems on the patient's quality of life:

- You need to explore the patient's perception of the severity of her acne. What makes her think that her skin has got worse recently?
- What effect is her acne having on her work? Any time off work?
- What is the effect on her general functioning? Has her acne affected her confidence levels?
- Has she stopped doing things – like going out socializing – because of her acne?
- Has anyone else – family, friends or work colleagues – commented on her skin?
- What are her own beliefs about the cause of her acne?
- What are her particular worries about the acne?
- What is her general mood like?
- Apart from the referral, was there anything else she wanted to happen as a result of seeing the doctor today?

Identifying a hidden agenda

The GP curriculum states that you need to be aware how cosmetic skin changes can affect a patient's interpersonal relationships. This patient will not offer the information about her boyfriend leaving her – and her belief that her skin was a cause of this – unless you tease this out:

- Why has she decided to attend today?
- Has anything happened recently – any major life events – that have prompted her to come back before her routine review appointment scheduled for 6–8 weeks?
- Once you have discovered that she believes her boyfriend left her because of her acne, you need sensitively to explore her reasons for thinking this.
- Has she been focusing on her acne as a way of avoiding confronting the reasons why her relationship ended? Giving her an opportunity to express her thoughts and feelings about what has happened may, in itself, prove therapeutic and help her to see her skin problem in perspective.

Domain 2 – Data gathering, examination and clinical assessment skills

Data gathering

Although you are told that the patient only has mild acne you still need to take a careful history:

- When did her acne first cause her problems? How have things progressed?
- How does she think things are now compared to when she came on the two previous visits 10 days ago and 10 months ago?
- What has she tried for her skin – including over-the-counter (OTC) and other people's medications? Has anything helped? Does anything make her acne worse?
- Any beliefs about her diet or cleanliness affecting her acne? The GP curriculum says that you should challenge and try and modify any false beliefs around skin problems.
- Is she taking any medication? The progesterone-only pill, topical steroids and phenytoin can all make acne worse.
- Is she aware that she should have been taking additional contraceptive precautions over the last 10 days? The BNF states that doxycycline may reduce the efficacy of combined oral contraceptives. However, if the antibiotic course exceeds 3 weeks, then additional precautions become unnecessary unless a new antibiotic is prescribed.
- Does she have flare ups of her acne which correspond to her periods? Any excessive hair? Any other signs of excess androgens?
- Is she applying topical medication properly – i.e. to all affected areas, not just to spots.
- She thinks that her acne is bad, but objectively it appears only mild. Does she have any other disproportionate concerns about her body – e.g. weight or shape?

Domain 3 – Clinical management skills

Dealing with a referral request

You are required to demonstrate a flexible approach to decision-making which incorporates a patient-centred approach. However, the GP curriculum also states that you should recognize the risk of inappropriate referrals:

- Why does she think she needs to see a specialist?
- Has she ever seen a skin specialist before?
- She has only tried oral antibiotics for 10 days and NICE guidelines suggest a minimum of two trials of oral antibiotics before referral to a specialist. Perhaps she could give the current treatment more time?
- She wants to be referred to have isotretinoin (Roaccutane), but does she know that this medication can be prescribed by a GP as a topical preparation? Would she be prepared to consider this?
- She is right that oral isotretinoin (Roaccutane) is only prescribed by a dermatologist, due to the risk of teratogenicity. However, does she understand

that this is usually considered only after other treatment options have failed or when there are signs of severe acne? Will she accept reassurance from you that her acne is only mild?

- One of the criteria for referral to specialist skin services is psychological distress. Although this patient is upset about breaking up with her boyfriend recently and is worried about her skin affecting her work, she does not appear unduly distressed or psychologically debilitated and there appear to be more appropriate options to try first before considering referral.

Reaching a shared management plan (overlap with Domain I)

This patient wants to be referred, but you could offer her a number of other management options:

- It is always worth giving simple advice such as:
  ○ Do not pick or squeeze spots.
  ○ Do not wash excessively and do not use exfoliating agents.
  ○ Do not use other people's medication – especially steroid cream.
- How would she feel about trying benzoyl peroxide again? It seemed to help her previously.
- Has she thought about giving the antibiotics longer to work? You could explain that we usually wait 3 months before considering switching to another oral antibiotic and she has only been taking the medication for 10 days.
- What does she think about the option of a topical retinoid, which she has not yet tried? If she does want to proceed, then you need to advise her that it can cause skin irritation initially and is contraindicated in pregnancy. She would also need to avoid exposure to UV light – e.g. apply sunscreen when outdoors and not use sun-beds or sun-lamps.
- There is also the option to combine the oral and topical treatments above – what does she think?
- You might be considering co-cyprindiol (Dianette) as an alternative to her combined oral contraceptive pill. However, the BNF states that this is licensed for use only in women with severe acne who have not responded to oral antibacterials and for moderately severe hirsutism.
- A referral at this stage would seem inappropriate. You need to explain to the patient in a rational and empathetic manner why this is the case and present her with a number of alternative options as outlined above.

Knowledge-base – Management of acne

References – BNF, NHS Clinical Knowledge Summaries.

Mild to moderate	*Topical*	<ul><li>Benzoyl peroxide<ul><li>Available OTC</li><li>Bactericidal</li><li>Consider when inflammatory lesions present</li></ul></li><li>Antibiotics – e.g. erythromycin, clindamycin, tetracycline</li><li>Retinoids<ul><li>E.g. tretinoin and isotretinoin</li><li>Consider in comedonal acne</li></ul></li></ul>Combined treatments – combining any two of the three above increases efficacy Azelaic acid – alternative to retinoids and benzoyl peroxide if neither tolerated
Moderate to severe	*Oral*	In addition to above, consider:<ul><li>Antibiotics<ul><li>E.g. first-line: tetracycline, oxytetracycline, doxycycline, lymecycline. Second-line: minocycline, erythromycin (latter if tetracycline contraindicated)</li><li>Consider if topical Rx has failed or there is moderate acne on the back or shoulders</li><li>Consider if inflammatory lesions present (risk of scarring)</li></ul></li></ul>
Severe and unresponsive to above	*Oral*	In addition to above, consider:<ul><li>Isotretinoin<ul><li>Prescribed only in secondary care</li><li>FBC, lipids, LFTs and negative pregnancy test before Rx</li><li>Contraception for minimum of 4 weeks before Rx</li><li>Needs careful monitoring as teratogenic</li></ul></li><li>Trimethoprim<ul><li>Dermatologist may consider as alternative antibiotic</li><li>Causes a rash in 5% of patients</li></ul></li></ul>

If a hormonal cause is likely, a combined oral contraceptive or co-cyprindiol (Dianette) may be appropriate.

Referral to a dermatologist is recommended if:

- Poor treatment response
- Scarring or pigmentation
- Nodulocystic acne
- Acne associated with psychological distress.

Take home messages

- Always consider why a patient has presented with their problem now – what in particular has triggered their attendance today?
- When a patient attends with inappropriate referral requests, attempt to offer alternative constructive management options.

Ideas for further revision

Referral requests can arise in many different CSA scenarios and can present a challenge to candidates. Look at other scenarios in this book and imagine that a request for a referral has been made. How would you deal with each of these requests in a sensitive yet appropriate manner?

Further reading

Acne Support Group. www.stopspots.org.

British Association of Dermatologists. www.bad.org.uk – includes patient information leaflets and management guidelines.

British National Formulary (BNF) www.bnf.org. Published jointly by BMJ Publishing Group and RPS Publishing, London. Updated every 6 months.

Dermatology Online Atlas. http://dermis.multimedica.de/index_e.html – image atlases with diagnoses and differential diagnoses.

NICE (2001) Referral advice – a guide to appropriate referral from general to specialist services. www.nice.org.uk.

NHS National Library for Health Clinical Knowledge Summaries – acne vulgaris. www.cks.library.nhs.uk/clinical_knowledge.

Primary Care Dermatology Society www.pcds.org.uk – includes guidelines and recommendations on primary care dermatology.

Examination 1: Station 5

Information given to candidates

David Foster is a 54-year-old company director with a past medical history of hypertension for which he takes a β-blocker – atenolol 25 mg OD – and a calcium channel blocker – amlodipine 10 mg OD. His hypertension has been well controlled for several years and the last reading when he saw the nurse 2 days ago was 128/80.

His records show that he is a smoker and drinks approximately 42 units of alcohol a week.

When he rang up to request an appointment, Mr Foster was offered the chance to see a nurse practitioner but requested to see a doctor to discuss a 'sensitive' issue.

You know that the patient's wife sees one of your colleagues in the practice and that she is being treated for depression.

When the patient first enters the room and sits down he says, "It's a bit embarrassing doctor, but I'm finding it difficult to have sex with my wife."

Assume that physical examination today is normal (including abdomen, genitals, prostate, pulse, BP, peripheral pulses and neurology) and that urinalysis is negative.

- What do you think this station is testing?
- Make notes or discuss your thoughts with a colleague before you read on.

Plan your approach to this station

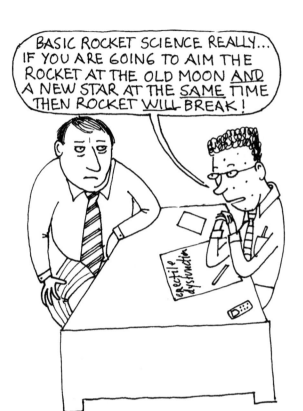

Information given to simulated patient

Basic details – You are David Foster, a Caucasian 54-year-old married man and company director.

Appearance and behaviour – You are smartly dressed and articulate, although you are embarrassed and find it hard to discuss the problem for which you have attended today – namely, impotence (also known as erectile dysfunction).

History

Freely divulged to doctor – You are finding it hard to get and maintain an erection to have sex with your wife. This has never been a problem for you in the past. You know that you want to have sex but 'things just don't seem to be working down below'. This is causing arguments between you and your wife. You moved into the spare room 2 days ago at your wife's request.

Divulged to doctor if specifically asked – You had an affair with a female colleague which lasted for 3 months. You ended this relationship 6 months ago as you realized that you had made a terrible mistake and still loved your wife. You have been married for 30 years and have never been unfaithful before. When the affair ended you told your wife what had happened and how you deeply regretted what you had done. Initially you moved out of the house for a month, but since then you have been back at home 'trying to make the relationship work'. You still find your wife sexually attractive. You and your wife have tried to have sex on four or five occasions since you moved back in, but you either cannot get any sort of erection, or your penis only gets semi-erect – not enough for sexual intercourse. You have never used condoms with your wife. You have woken with a full erection on several occasions and you have been able to obtain and maintain an erection for masturbation when you have been alone. When you have masturbated you had no problems ejaculating. Last night on an impulse you went round to the house of the woman you had the affair with and ended up having sex. You deeply regret your actions. You did not have any problems getting or maintaining an erection for intercourse with her. You have not had any discharge from your penis, or any genital irritation. You have never had any sexually transmitted infections. You are not excessively thirsty. You do not have any genital pain. You have not felt depressed or particularly stressed recently. You have not had any other symptoms such as chest pain, leg pain or numbness.

Ideas, concerns and expectations – You feel guilty about being unfaithful to your wife – especially your actions last night – and also because you think the recent bout of depression that your wife has been suffering from was triggered by telling her about the affair. You are hoping that the doctor can 'check you out' to make sure there are no problems 'down below', although you suspect that the problem is 'in your head'. You used condoms when you had sex with your colleague during the affair and last night, but part of you thinks that you could still have picked something up that you could pass on to your wife. You checked the information leaflets for your blood pressure tablets and saw that sexual dysfunction was listed as a side effect for both drugs. You have kept taking the medication but you want to ask the doctor about this.

First words spoken to doctor – "It's a bit embarrassing doctor, but I'm finding it difficult to have sex with my wife."

Past medical history – You were diagnosed with high blood pressure 4 years ago, but your blood pressure has been fine on the tablets. You see the practice nurse every 6 months to get your blood pressure checked.

Drug history – You have been taking two different tablets for your blood pressure for over 3 years: atenolol 25 mg one tablet once a day and amlodipine 10 mg one tablet once a day. You have not tried any medication to help with your impotence. You are not allergic to any medication.

Social history – You are a director in a successful technology company, which makes circuit boards for mobile phones. You smoke one or two cigars a day. You smoked about 20 cigarettes a day from when you were in your 20s until 10 years ago, when you switched to cigars. You drink a very generous glass of whiskey most days and a couple of glasses of wine with your evening meal.

Family history – There are no major medical problems in your immediate family.

- Having read the information given to the simulated patient, what do you now think this station is testing?
- Make notes or discuss your thoughts with a colleague before you turn the page.

Review your approach to this station:

Tested at this station:

1. Dealing with a sensitive topic
2. Data gathering
3. Taking a sexual history
4. Reaching a shared management plan

Domain 1 – Interpersonal skills

Dealing with a sensitive topic

The new GP curriculum points out that male genitourinary problems are increasing and men are often embarrassed to present with these conditions. This patient is clearly uncomfortable in discussing his erectile dysfunction. You need to try and put the patient at ease by being both empathic and professional:

- Acknowledge his discomfort at having to discuss such a personal matter.
- Explain that such problems are common and that he has made a significant first step in coming to see you today.
- Before you begin taking a history explain that problems such as his can have physical and psychological causes – and are often a combination of the two – so that he understands your rationale for asking specific questions.
- Take some time to explore his ideas, concerns and expectations – he feels guilty at having the affair and particularly over his actions last night. Taking time now to enquire about these issues should elicit key facts and emotions that will help you identify and address his agenda.
- Discussing sexual matters can be difficult even for healthcare professionals, but if the patient senses any unease or embarrassment on your part, then this will compound his discomfort.
- You may have strong personal beliefs about adultery, but you need to remain professional and non-judgemental during the consultation.

Domain 2 – Data gathering, examination and clinical assessment skills

Data gathering

Taking a detailed general history will help you identify the probable cause(s) of his erectile dysfunction:

- How long have the erection problems been going on for?
- Any triggers?
- Any previous difficulty getting or maintaining an erection?
- Any previous pelvic surgery?
- Does he have excessive thirst, dysuria, urinary frequency or nocturia?
- Any numbness, weakness, reduced sensation or visual problems?
- Does he suffer from chest pain, pain in his legs when he walks or previous heart or circulation problems?
- Is he able to get an erection if he masturbates? Any problems with ejaculation?

- Does he ever wake up with an erection?
- How has his mood been recently? Is he under particular stress at work?
- How much alcohol does he drink?
- Does he smoke?

Taking a sexual history

Although you will have covered some of the issues around his erectile dysfunction in the general history, it is important not to shy away from taking a specific sexual history for anyone who presents with genital symptoms. In this case, failure to take a detailed sexual history would result in missing a key fact that the patient managed to have intercourse last night with his colleague, without any erectile dysfunction:

- Signpost the fact that you need to ask some further personal questions about his sexual activity, to help reach a diagnosis. Explain that you ask the same questions of everyone who has these sorts of problems.
- When was the last time he had sex?
- Who was it with? Was it with his wife or with another partner? Was the partner male or female (if this is not immediately obvious from his previous response)?
- Did they use condoms?
- When did he have sex prior to that episode? – If this was with a different partner, then ask the same set of questions as above.
- Has he had any sexually transmitted infections (STIs) in the past?
- Any penile discharge?

Physical examination

Patients presenting with erectile dysfunction should normally be examined to look for hypogonadism (e.g. small or absent testes), secondary sexual characteristics (e.g. gynaecomastia), any signs of penile discharge and structural deformities (e.g. Peyronie disease). For this station you have been informed that a comprehensive physical examination – including abdomen, genitals, prostate, pulse, BP, peripheral pulses and neurology – together with urinalysis, are normal.

Domain 3 – Clinical management skills

Reaching a shared management plan (overlap with Domain I)

As this is a particularly sensitive topic, you need to ensure that any management plan is one which the patient feels comfortable with and has been negotiated to both parties' satisfaction:

- The patient is worried that he may have 'picked something up' through having sex with a different partner. You can reassure him that using condoms greatly reduces the chance of acquiring STIs. But has he considered getting a sexual health check at the local genitourinary medicine clinic? This might put his mind at rest regarding having an STI.

- He is concerned that his erectile dysfunction may be related to his blood pressure tablets. Given that he has been taking these for 3 years, had not experienced any impotence prior to his affair, and was able to have intercourse last night, you could explain that the tablets are unlikely to be the main cause of his current problems. However, if he wishes to try alternative medication this would always be an option, although switching drugs could temporarily disturb his otherwise excellent blood pressure control.
- His alcohol intake is excessive – has he considered trying to cut down on his drinking? This could make a significant difference to his erectile problems.
- You can explain that given the history and the normal physical examination there seems to be a large psychological component to his inability to get a full erection with his wife. How does he feel about this suggestion?
- What does he think about couple counselling, such as through Relate? Would his wife be willing to participate?
- Explain that there are other 'talking therapies' that may help, such as psychosexual counselling.
- Although his problems have a strong psychological component, given his history of smoking, alcohol consumption and high blood pressure, you may wish to discuss doing some routine tests to look at his cholesterol level, blood glucose, LFTs and kidney function. Other blood tests to exclude a physical component to his erectile dysfunction could include PSA and testosterone (morning sample). If the testosterone level is low, then prolactin, FSH and LH blood tests should also be taken.
- Praise the fact that he cut down from 20 cigarettes a day to one or two cigars. But is he ready to give up completely? This would have a beneficial effect on his general health as well as helping prevent his erectile problems from worsening.
- Explain that there are tablets which can help with erectile dysfunction (see below), but as he does not experience any problems except with his wife, it is probably best first to explore the psychological aspect through counselling. What does he think?
- Arrange to see him in a couple of weeks for follow-up, to discuss the results of any blood tests and to see how things are progressing.

Knowledge-base – Erectile dysfunction (ED)

References – BNF and see Further reading.

Causes – may be multifactorial	Details	Management
Psychogenic	• Generalized (e.g. lack of arousability) or situational (e.g. partner-related) • Usually presents as sudden onset of ED	• Psychosexual counselling • Sensate focused therapy (stroking only initially: non-genitals, then genitals, then intercourse – therapist gives permission for progression) • Treatments for ED as below may be of benefit
Vascular	• Atherosclerosis leading to impaired blood flow to the penis • A detailed cardiovascular history should elicit clues • Usually presents as gradual onset of ED	• Stop smoking if applicable • Assess for other signs of cardiovascular disease (CVD) • Treat modifiable CVD risk factors aggressively (e.g. lifestyle, BP, cholesterol) • Treatments for ED as below may be of benefit
Neurological	• Multiple sclerosis • Parkinson's disease • Stroke • Spinal injury • Cauda equina syndrome • Post surgical (e.g. prostatectomy)	• Treat neurological condition appropriately • Treatments for ED as below may be of benefit
Endocrine	• Diabetes mellitus • Thyroid dysfunction • Hypogonadism • Hyperprolactinaemia	• Urinalysis for glucose and serum glucose • TFTs. Treat any thyroid disease appropriately • Check testosterone levels. Testosterone injections may be indicated • Check prolactin if testosterone levels low
Drug induced	• Excessive alcohol consumption • Antihypertensive medication of all classes, most common are diuretics and β-blockers • Antidepressants • Antipsychotics • Antihistamines • Antiandrogens • H$_2$ antagonists	• Reduce alcohol intake • If possible, switch medication to alternatives which do not have ED as a side effect

- First-line pharmacotherapy for ED (once 'curable' causes such as testosterone deficiency have been excluded) includes phosphodiesterase type 5 inhibitors such as sildenafil, tadalafil and vardenafil. These treat ED by increasing blood flow to the penis.
- Such drugs for ED can only be prescribed on the NHS if the patient has diabetes, multiple sclerosis, Parkinson's disease, poliomyelitis, prostate cancer, severe pelvic injury, spina bifida, spinal cord injury or single gene neurological disease; is on dialysis for renal failure; has had radical pelvic surgery, prostatectomy or kidney transplant; is suffering severe distress (must be prescribed in this case by a specialist centre); or was receiving treatment for ED on the NHS on 14th September 1998.
- Other treatments for ED include sublingual apomorphine, intracavernosal alprostadil injections, intraurethral alprostadil, vacuum devices and penile prostheses.

Take home messages

- Erectile dysfunction is a common condition that can cause patients significant embarrassment.
- A professional and empathetic approach is essential for such consultations.
- When dealing with sensitive issues such as erectile dysfunction, it is all the more important to involve patients in management options to optimise concordance.

Ideas for further revision

Although the CSA is primarily an assessment of skills, there will be times when simulated patients put candidates on the spot by asking for a specific piece of factual knowledge. For example, *"How does that drug work, doctor?"* or *"But do I have to tell the DVLA about my condition?"* Given that both the CSA and the Applied Knowledge Test (AKT) are offered three times a year, you might find it useful to sit both assessments together, so that you can integrate your revision.

Further reading

American Urology Association: Management of Erectile Dysfunction (updated 2006). www.auanet.org/guidelines/edmgmt.cfm.

British National Formulary (BNF). Published jointly by BMJ Publishing Group and RPS Publishing, London. Updated every 6 months. www.bnf.org.

European Association of Urology: Guidelines on erectile dysfunction (updated March 2005). www.library.nhs.uk/guidelinesfinder/ViewResource.aspx?resID=143318.

Patient UK has clinical summaries specifically designed for doctors – e.g. erectile dysfunction. www.patient.co.uk/showdoc/40000959/.

Sexual Dysfunction Association offers information and support for those who suffer from erectile dysfunction, premature or delayed ejaculation, and Peyronie disease. On-line information for patients can be found at www.sda.uk.net.

Wakley G, Cunnion M, Chambers R. *Improving Sexual Health Advice*. Oxford: Radcliffe Medical Press, 2003.

Information given to candidates

> Amy Richards is a 56-year-old who has been with the practice for over 20 years.
>
> She has been taking levothyroxine 75 μg OD for 8 years. She has regular blood tests monitoring her TFTs, which have been stable for several years.
>
> Otherwise she attends the surgery only occasionally with minor self-limiting illnesses.
>
> Her records show that she is often prescribed antibiotics on these occasions.
>
> You note that she normally sees the senior partner when she attends the surgery.

As the patient enters the consultation room she says, "I need some antibiotics for this ear infection."

If you perform otoscopy during the consultation, assume that you find no abnormality in either ear.

- What do you think this station is testing?
- Make notes or discuss your thoughts with a colleague before you read on.

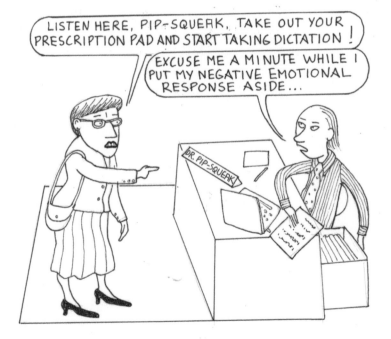

Plan your approach to this station:

Information given to simulated patient

Basic details – You are Amy Richards, a Caucasian 56-year-old single woman who works in the local council's finance department.

Appearance and behaviour – You come across as rather demanding.

History
Freely divulged to doctor – Yesterday evening your left ear started aching. This kept you awake much of the night and you have not been able to go into work today because of the pain. You took two paracetamol tablets last night, but thought you would wait to see the doctor before taking any more pills. Your right ear is fine. You want some antibiotics for your 'ear infection'.

Divulged to doctor if specifically asked – You have had a cold, with a runny nose and sore throat for 3 days. Since last night the hearing in your left ear has been a little muffled. You have not noticed any discharge from your ears. Your balance has been fine. You have not had any episodes of dizziness or sensations of spinning. You had a similar 'ear infection' last year for which the senior partner gave you antibiotics (you cannot remember the name of the medication), and this seemed to clear things up within a couple of days.

Ideas, concerns and expectations –You are frustrated at not being able to see the senior partner, who you used to go to school with, and usually see for consultations. You think that antibiotics will help your ear problem, as they seemed to do so before. You will find it hard to accept if the doctor says that antibiotics are not immediately indicated – if the senior partner prescribed them before, why is a more junior doctor saying something different today? But you may be persuaded if the doctor treats your concerns with respect and adequately explains your diagnosis and what the best treatment options are.

First words spoken to doctor – "I need some antibiotics for this ear infection."

Past medical history – You have an under-active thyroid gland and take medication for this daily. You attend the surgery for regular blood tests to check your thyroid hormones levels. These have been fine and your medication dose has remained the same for over 4 years. Otherwise you come to the surgery occasionally with coughs, colds and minor illnesses, for which you often receive antibiotics.

Drug history – You have been taking levothyroxine 75 µg once a day for 8 years. You are allergic to penicillin – your mother told you that you got a nasty rash and 'swelled up' when you had penicillin as a child.

Social history – You live on your own in a terraced house. You have never smoked and drink a glass or two of wine with your evening meal. You grew up near the GP surgery and have lived and worked in the area ever since. You have an active social life, centred around the local amateur dramatics society.

Family history – Your mother died of breast cancer when she was 88 years old. You have two younger brothers who are fit and well.

- Having read the information given to the simulated patient, what do you now think this station is testing?
- Make notes or discuss your thoughts with a colleague before you turn the page.

Review your approach to this station:

Tested at this station:

1. Dealing with a demanding patient
2. History taking skills
3. Physical examination skills
4. Management of common medical conditions presenting in primary care

Domain I – Interpersonal skills

Dealing with a demanding patient

Some patients seem to know exactly what they want, and during the consultation can come across as demanding. This may invoke negative emotional responses in you that need to be recognized and placed to one side if you are going to manage the consultation in a positive and constructive manner:

- This patient has stated right at the outset what she wants you to do. Acknowledging her request is a good starting point.
- Often patients can appear demanding if they are unhappy about some aspect of their care – e.g. if they have been kept waiting or had problems getting an appointment. In this case the patient wanted to see the senior partner. If you can elicit such issues – e.g. by asking if there have been any problems with coming to see you today – then you can help defuse any potential conflict in the consultation.
- Why does she believe that she needs antibiotics? How do her previous experiences inform her current demands?
- What are her worries if she does not have her request met?
- If she insists on demanding a certain course of action – such as antibiotics – you might try explaining the rationale for current best practice – e.g. how we now believe that taking antibiotics for mild, self-limiting infections can increase antibiotic resistance, is unlikely significantly to help recovery and risks causing unpleasant side effects such as vomiting, diarrhoea and a rash. What does she think about this?
- In this case, the patient has certain expectations in light of her previous consultations. If you refuse to meet her demands today she may simply re-book to see the senior partner who – given his track record – could undermine your actions by prescribing antibiotics to the patient. The scope of the CSA includes problem-solving skills and these are meant to include – among other things – being able to adopt a flexible approach to decision-making.

Domain 2 – Data gathering, examination and clinical assessment skills

History taking skills

Although ear pain presenting in primary care is commonly a symptom of a minor, self-limiting illness, it is important to take an adequate history to help rule out more serious diagnoses and guide antibiotic prescribing decisions:

- Is one or are both ears affected?
- Are her ears painful?

- Any discharge?
- Has she noticed any problem with her hearing?
- Any sensation of ringing in her ears (tinnitus)?
- Any problems with her balance or sensations of movement, such as spinning?
- Has she had any other symptoms recently, such as a cough or runny nose?
- Has she been feverish or vomited?
- Any previous ear problems?
- What work does she do? Any exposure through work to potential causes of ear problems? – e.g. swimming instructor, exposure to loud noise at work.
- Any other pains in her head or neck?
- What medication is she taking? – certain drugs can be ototoxic, such as furosemide.

Physical examination skills

When a patient complains of ear pain or problems with their hearing, a proficient physical examination is required as part of your overall assessment:

- Otoscopy – explain to the patient what will be involved and gain consent before proceeding with the examination:
  - If the patient presents with a problem in one ear, always start by examining the other 'good' ear first.
  - In adults, pulling the pinna backwards and upwards during otoscopy helps straighten out the canal and allows better visualization of the tympanic membrane.
  - Start by examining the pinna and external auditory meatus for debris, discharge or lesions.
  - Examine the external auditory canal for signs of inflammation, swelling, excessive wax or foreign bodies.
  - Can you visualize the tympanic membrane? What colour is it? Any signs of bulging or retraction? Is there an appropriate light reflex? Can you see a fluid level behind the tympanic membrane?
  - If you see a perforation centrally, then this is considered safe. However, if the perforation is marginal then it may indicate cholesteatoma and requires referral.
  - Always review patients if you cannot see the tympanic membrane.
- Hearing assessment – in the GP surgery a simple whisper test is adequate for gross hearing assessment. Ask the patient to repeat whispered words with distraction in the other ear by rubbing the tragus.
- Tuning fork tests (512 Hz) – Rinne's and Weber's tests are indicated if the history suggests hearing loss:
  - *Rinne's test* – place the vibrating tuning fork against the bone just behind the patient's ear. Then move the tuning folk beside the external auditory meatus. Ask her which is louder. If the patient's hearing is normal, or if there is sensorineural hearing loss in that ear, then the sound should be louder next to the meatus (air conduction greater than bone conduction). If she has conductive hearing loss (or severe sensorineural hearing loss) in that ear, then she will hear the sound louder behind the ear.

○ *Weber's test* – place the vibrating tuning fork in the middle of the patient's forehead and ask her where she can hear the sound – in the middle or to one side. If she hears the sound to one side, it suggests conductive hearing loss on that side or sensorineural hearing loss on the other side.

Domain 3 – Clinical management skills

Management of common medical conditions presenting in primary care

You need to feel confident at recognizing and managing common ENT problems presenting in primary care. The GP curriculum states that you should demonstrate an evidence-based approach to antibiotic prescribing – e.g. in otitis media – to prevent antibiotic resistance:

- You can reassure the patient that examination of her ears shows no signs of any serious infection.
- Does she understand that symptoms of a mild ear infection usually resolve within 3 days without antibiotics?
- Is she prepared to consider 'watchful waiting' as a management option?
- You could reinforce how she has done the right thing in taking painkillers, and advise that self-medication with regular paracetamol and ibuprofen will help her symptoms.
- Delayed antibiotic prescribing – where a prescription is collected by the patient after 3 days if symptoms are not improving or earlier if symptoms worsen. This represents another option which may be acceptable to the patient. What does she think about this?
- If you are going to prescribe, remember to ask about allergies – this patient is allergic to penicillin.
- Referral to audiology would be indicated if you had any concern regarding hearing loss.
- This consultation is also an opportunity for patient education regarding self-management of minor self-limiting illnesses and alternatives to seeing the doctor – such as asking the pharmacist or NHS Direct for advice.

Knowledge-base – Ear infections

References – NHS Clinical Knowledge Summaries, MeReC Bulletin.

General	• Ear infections can occur at any age, but are more common in children

Otitis media	• Inflammation of the middle ear
	• Acute otitis media (AOM) versus otitis media with effusion (OME) – glue ear:
	  ○ AOM – often preceded by upper respiratory symptoms (cough, runny nose). Rapid onset. Can present with ear pain, fever, poor sleep, irritability. Signs may include cloudy, bulging or distinctly red or immobile tympanic membrane
	  ○ OME – often asymptomatic. Children can present with hearing problems or speech delay, secondary to chronic inflammation and build up of fluid within middle ear

Acute otitis media (AOM)	• Can be viral or bacterial in origin • Is usually a self-limiting illness – resolves within 3 days without antibiotics in majority of patients • Rare complications include mastoiditis, labyrinthitis and meningitis

Treatment for AOM	• Use of decongestants or antihistamines have insufficient evidence base
	• Simple analgesics – paracetamol and ibuprofen – can help relieve pain and fever
	• Antibiotics have been shown to have a modest beneficial effect on the risk of pain after 2 days – 7% absolute risk reduction. But given the risks of side effects and antibiotic resistance, they are not recommended routinely for the treatment of AOM
	• Antibiotics may be indicated if patients have:
	  ○ Systemic features – e.g. vomiting or high fever
	  ○ Recurrent infections
	  ○ A discharging ear
	  ○ Bilateral ear infections
	  ○ Under 2 years old
	• Where antibiotics are indicated, amoxicillin is considered first-line treatment (5 day course: < 2 years 125 mg TDS; 2–10 years 250 mg TDS; > 10 years 500 mg TDS). Erythromycin can be used for patients allergic to penicillin – as in this scenario – but it is less effective against *Haemophilus influenzae*. Azithromycin and clarithromycin can also be used
	• Delayed prescribing – prescription to be collected by patient after 3 days if symptoms are not improving or earlier if symptoms worsen – helps reduce antibiotic use and re-attendance rates

Take home messages

- Understanding and acknowledging a patient's concerns can help defuse potential conflict when they present with demands for treatment.
- The CSA is not just designed to test consultation skills – you must demonstrate proficiency in physical examinations, too.

Ideas for further revision

Patient education, including advising on the appropriate use of healthcare resources, is a key role of the GP. In your day-to-day practice, do not shy away from such discussions, but instead look to inform patients of the various sources of healthcare advice and support available, which may be more readily accessible, and more appropriate, than booking to see their GP.

Further reading

BMJ Topic collections ENT references. www.bmj.com/cgi/collection/otolaryngology.

MeReC Bulletin – The Management of Common Infections in Primary Care. Volume 17, Number 3. December 2006 – section on acute otitis media. www.npc.co.uk/MeReC_Bulletins/MeReC_Bulletin_Vol17_No3_Intro.htm.

NHS National Library for Health Clinical Knowledge Summaries – otitis media. www.cks.library.nhs.uk/clinical_knowledge.

Information given to candidates

> You are a salaried GP, employed by a practice whose senior partner is Dr Mickle. You have worked with Dr Mickle for over a year. He is a competent doctor but under some stress at the moment because of a difficult divorce.
>
> Emily Johnson, one of the nurse practitioners, has asked to see you to discuss a patient, Shen Li. She explained in an email that she is concerned with the management of this patient by Dr Mickle.
>
> Mr Li's notes state that he is a 42-year-old builder who has been complaining of feeling tired for several months. His fasting blood glucose results are recorded as:
>
> 7.8 mmol/L – 2 weeks ago
> 8.4 mmol/L – last week

As she enters the consultation room Emily Johnson says, "Doctor you must do something. Dr Mickle is a liability to this practice – he's unsafe as a doctor and extremely rude to colleagues and patients."

- What do you think this station is testing?
- Make notes or discuss your thoughts with a colleague before you read on.

Plan your approach to this station:

Information given to simulated colleague

Basic details – You are Emily Johnson, a Caucasian 48-year-old nurse practitioner working in a GP surgery. You are qualified to see patients on your own and to manage a range of medical conditions presenting in primary care.

Appearance and behaviour – You are upset and angry at how you have been treated by the senior partner, Dr Mickle. But if the doctor you see today is empathetic and understanding, then you will become more composed.

History

Freely divulged to doctor – You saw a patient – Shen Li – 3 weeks ago with an uncomplicated ear infection. During the consultation he said that he had been feeling tired for several months. You arranged for him to see the practice phlebotomist to have some routine blood tests, including thyroid function tests and a fasting blood glucose. These were normal apart from a raised glucose – at 7.8 mmol/L. You telephoned the patient and asked him to book to see one of the doctors to discuss the results. The patient asked you on the telephone whether there was anything to worry about and you said that he would need to discuss things with the doctor, but that he probably had diabetes.

Divulged to doctor if specifically asked – You next saw the patient 3 days ago. He told you that – as requested – he had seen Dr Mickle who had said that it was necessary to repeat the blood glucose test. The patient told you that he had had the second blood test and gone back to see Dr Mickle for the result. (You checked this result on the computer and it was 8.4 mmol/L.) According to the patient, Dr Mickle said that his results were nothing to worry about, but that it was important to keep an eye on his blood sugar levels by doing another blood test in 6 months. Mr Li wanted to complain to you about Dr Mickle's manner, saying that Dr Mickle had been dismissive and rude when he (Mr Li) had asked whether he had diabetes. You found this meeting with the patient very difficult as he kept asking why you had said that he had diabetes but Dr Mickle said that he did not. The following day you tried to discuss the matter with Dr Mickle, but Dr Mickle got angry and said that you were not medically qualified and should not be questioning his clinical judgement. Your relationship with Dr Mickle has been a little strained for some time, ever since you felt that he had blocked your suggestions for developing the minor illness service at the surgery last year. You do not know about any other incidents with patients where Dr Mickle's management has given any cause for concern. Dr Mickle seems to have been rather short-tempered this last month and has had several days off for illness recently – which is quite unlike him. You told the patient that you would discuss the matter with Dr Mickle and see the patient again to try and answer his questions about his diagnosis.

Ideas, concerns and expectations – You think that Dr Mickle has missed the diagnosis of diabetes mellitus in the patient Shen Li. You do not understand why he would have made this error. You do not really think that he is 'unsafe as a doctor', but you are upset about how he has behaved towards you. You did not like being made to look stupid and you are worried that relations with Dr Mickle – who is the senior partner and your employer – have deteriorated further. You do want to try and resolve the situation, and hope that the doctor you are seeing today will be able somehow to 'sort out this mess'. You would be happy to attend a meeting with Dr Mickle, if someone else were there to give you support. You would also be happy if the doctor wants to discuss things first with Dr Mickle on his own, or to seek advice from others on how best to proceed.

First words spoken to doctor – "Doctor you must do something. Dr Mickle is a liability to this practice – he's unsafe as a doctor and extremely rude to colleagues and patients."

Past medical history – You are fit and well and have never suffered from any significant medical problems.

Drug history – You do not take any regular medication.

Social history – You work full-time at the GP surgery and live with your husband and teenage son.

Family history – There are no significant medical problems in your immediate family.

- Having read the information given to the simulated colleague, what do you now think this station is testing?
- Make notes or discuss your thoughts with a colleague before you turn the page.

Review your approach to this station:

Tested at this station:

1. Providing support to a colleague
2. Gathering information in relation to a complaint
3. Dealing with a complaint about a colleague
4. Understanding patient safety issues

Domain 1 – Interpersonal skills

Providing support to a colleague

One of your colleagues is visibly distressed at events at work. She has chosen to speak to you about this matter and you need to be understanding and supportive in your response:

- Allow her freely to express her thoughts about what has happened. Use active listening skills to demonstrate your attentiveness, together with open questions to encourage her fully to disclose her perspective on events.
- Empathize with her situation and the stressful meetings she has had, both with the patient and Dr Mickle.
- Ask her what she was hoping you could do to help.
- If she wants to discuss the matter again with Dr Mickle, but would like someone else there for support, then you could offer to arrange the meeting and be present.

Domain 2 – Data gathering, examination and clinical assessment skills

Gathering information in relation to a complaint

After you have given the nurse practitioner an opportunity to tell her story, it is important to try and ascertain her precise account of events. More specific closed questions may help you in this regard:

- Can she tell you when she first thought there was a problem?
- Can she describe exactly what happened at each meeting with the patient? When did these take place?
- When she tried to discuss the matter with Dr Mickle what happened?
- What makes her say that Dr Mickle is 'unsafe as a doctor'? Have there been any other incidents involving Dr Mickle that she would like to discuss?
- She says that the patient told her that Dr Mickle was rude to him – can she say more about this? Has the patient made a formal complaint?
- Does she know who took the blood samples? Were they definitely fasting samples?
- What arrangements have been made with the patient for follow-up?

Domain 3 – Clinical management skills

Dealing with a complaint about a colleague

One of the members of your clinical team has made a complaint about another doctor you both work alongside. You need to take this seriously and act appropriately:

- As the GP curriculum makes clear, all health professionals are expected to adhere to ethical principles which are the framework for professional codes of conduct (see Knowledge-base and Further reading).
- These codes outline minimum standards of practice and limits to behaviour.
- The allegations put to you are that one of your medical colleagues:
  - Incorrectly reassured a patient that he did not have diabetes
  - Was rude and dismissive when the matter was raised with him by a fellow health professional
  - Was rude to the patient involved.
- According to the nurse practitioner, Dr Mickle's recent behaviour is out of character for him. There is also the suggestion that his health may be suffering – he has taken several days off sick recently, which is quite unlike him. His short temper and time off work could be related to his divorce. However, you should not divulge this personal information, although you could agree that he does appear to have been rather stressed recently.
- You cannot fully understand the situation without discussing the matter with Dr Mickle. For example, it may be that the blood tests were not in fact fasting samples, and this is why Dr Mickle has reassured the patient that he does not have diabetes. However, even if this turns out to be the case, there are still questions as to the professional behaviour of Dr Mickle towards his colleague and the patient.

Understanding patient safety issues

When a concern is raised about a colleague, your first priority must be to ascertain whether patients have been, or are likely to be, put at risk:

- You could make clear to the nurse practitioner that if a mistake has been made, then you would be happy to explain this to the patient, apologize and describe what steps will be taken to reduce the chance of this happening again. However, first you need to speak to Dr Mickle, both to gather more information and to offer him some support.
- As the Royal College of General Practice and the British Medical Association make clear (see Knowledge-base), when relationships within the healthcare team break down, patient care usually suffers. Therefore, from a patient safety perspective, it is important to try and resolve the dispute between the nurse practitioner and Dr Mickle.
- Reflective practice around patient safety issues is a key opportunity for staff and organizations to learn about, and improve, patient care. So it is important to have an open and constructive approach to discussing incidents where concerns have been raised about patient safety. One way forward would therefore be to propose a practice meeting to discuss the criteria for diagnosing diabetes.
- In summary, your options include:
  - Offering to arrange a meeting with Dr Mickle on his own.
  - Offering to arrange a meeting with Dr Mickle and the nurse practitioner.

○ Offering to see the patient, once you have ascertained further information about events.
○ Organizing a practice meeting reviewing criteria for diabetes diagnosis and perhaps suggesting a practice policy or guideline.

Knowledge-base

Professional and ethical issues

References – GMC guidance, RCGP and BMA guidance – see Further reading.

GMC *Good Medical Practice 2006*	Good doctors (para 1)	Good doctors make the care of their patients their first concern: they are competent, keep their knowledge up to date, establish and maintain good relationships with patients and colleagues, are honest and trustworthy, and act with integrity
	Working in teams (para 41)	When working in a team, you should act as a positive role model and try and motivate and inspire your colleagues. You must: respect the skills and contributions of your colleagues
	Conduct and performance of colleagues (para 43)	You must protect patients from risk of harm posed by another colleague's conduct, performance or health. The safety of patients must come first at all times. If you have concerns that a colleague may not be fit to practise, you must take appropriate steps without delay, so that the concerns are investigated and patients protected where necessary
	Respect for colleagues (para 46)	You must treat your colleagues fairly and with respect […] You should challenge colleagues if their behaviour does not comply with this guidance
RCGP and BMA *Good Medical Practice for General Practitioners 2002*	Working with colleagues and working in teams (section 11)	• Good team working includes respecting colleagues, both personally and professionally • When relationships within the team break down, patient care usually suffers. Therefore, ensuring good communication within your team is an important part of being a good GP
	Protecting patients when your own health or the health, conduct or performance of other doctors puts patients at risk (section 18)	The excellent GP: • Is aware when a colleague's performance, conduct, or health might be putting patients at risk • Quickly and discreetly ascertains the facts of the case, takes advice from colleagues, and, if appropriate, refers the colleague for medical advice or local remedial action • Provides positive support to colleagues who have made mistakes or whose performance gives cause for concern • You have a responsibility to do something if patients are being put at risk through poor performance or because the doctor is ill • You now risk an allegation of misconduct if you know a doctor is unsafe and you do nothing about it • If you are in doubt, take advice. Sometimes this will be from one of your partners. Outside the practice, you can talk to your Local Medical Committee chairman or secretary, or to your defense society

Diabetes mellitus diagnosis

Reference – WHO 1999 – see Further reading.

Diagnosis	*Findings*
Diabetes mellitus	Symptomatic ● With one random blood glucose ≥ 11.1 mmol/L ● With one fasting blood glucose ≥ 7.0 mmol/L
	Asymptomatic ● With two random blood glucose results on different days ≥ 11.1 mmol/L ● With two fasting blood glucose results on different days ≥ 7.0 mmol/L
	Glucose tolerance test – give 75 mg glucose to fasting patient, take sample after 2 h ● Blood glucose ≥ 11.1 mmol/L
Impaired fasting glycaemia	● Fasting blood glucose ≥ 6.1 mmol/L and < 7.0 mmol/L ● And (if measured) blood glucose < 7.8 mmol/L 2 h post glucose load in glucose tolerance test
Impaired glucose tolerance	Glucose tolerance test ● Blood glucose ≥ 7.8 mmol/L and < 11.1 mmol/L 2 h post glucose load

Take home messages

- You need to be aware of the professional ethical guidelines which are central to your practice as a GP.
- When patients or colleagues come to you with a complaint, you can be supportive and understanding without having to make an immediate judgement as to the merit of the complaint.
- Patient safety must always take priority.

Ideas for further revision

This station is primarily looking at relationships with colleagues and patient safety issues. However, it is important to be familiar with the diagnostic criteria for diabetes mellitus to help you in your response. Other CSA stations may focus on data interpretation in more detail and you should feel comfortable interpreting blood test results, child growth charts, cervical smear reports, spirometry graphs, imaging reports, ECGs, and other clinical test results that are commonly seen in general practice.

Further reading

Association of British Clinical Diabetologists. www.diabetologists-abcd.org.uk.

Department of Health. *An Organisation with a Memory*. London: The Stationery Office, 2000. www.dh.gov.uk/en/Publicationsandstatistics/Publications/PublicationsPolicyAndGuidance/DH_4065083.

Department of Health. *National Service Framework for Diabetes: Standards* (Department of Health, England), 2001. www.dh.gov.uk/PolicyAndGuidance/HealthAndSocialCareTopics/Diabetes/fs/en.

General Medical Council. *Good Medical Practice*. London: GMC, November 2006. www.gmc-uk.org/guidance/good_medical_practice/index.asp.

General Practitioners Committee of the BMA and the Royal College of General Practitioners. *Good Medical Practice for General Practitioners*. London: RCGP, 2002. www.rcgp.org.uk/PDF/Corp_GMP06.pdf.

National Patient Safety Agency. Being Open Policy, 2005. www.npsa.nhs.uk.

RCGP curriculum statements – Personal and Professional Responsibilities: 3.2 Patient Safety; 3.3 Clinical Ethics and Values-Based Practice. www.rcgp-curriculum.org.uk/curriculum_documents/gp_curriculum_statements.aspx.

World Health Organization (WHO). Definition, diagnosis and classification of diabetes mellitus and its complications, 1999. www.staff.ncl.ac.uk/philip.home/who_dmc.htm.

Information given to candidates

Wesley Anderson is a 58-year-old Black British man who rarely comes to the surgery.

He attended 3 months ago with a sprained right ankle, injured while playing football, which resolved with ibuprofen.

He had his BP routinely checked at that time and it was 156/98. Cardiovascular examination and fundoscopy were otherwise normal. He was given lifestyle advice.

He returned 6 weeks later to have his BP re-checked and was seen by a different GP. Cardiovascular examination and fundoscopy were again normal and his BP was 158/96. Urine dip-stick was normal. Various blood tests were requested. The patient was again given lifestyle advice to try and help him lower his BP.

He returned today and saw the nurse. His BP was 156/96 and he was asked to see the doctor to discuss his blood tests and BP.

FBC	Normal	Height	180 cm
U&Es	Normal	Weight	100.4 kg
LFTs	Normal	BMI	31 kg/m^2
Glucose	5.2 mmol/L		
Total cholesterol	6.0 mmol/L		
HDL	1.0 mmol/L		

As the patient enters the room he says, "The nurse said to see you to get the results of my blood tests and have a chat about my blood pressure."

On the desk in front of you are cardiovascular risk prediction charts (reproduced in the back of the BNF).

- What do you think this station is testing?
- Make notes or discuss your thoughts with a colleague before you read on.

Plan your approach to this station:

Information given to simulated patient

Basic details – You are Wesley Anderson, a 58-year-old Black British man who was born and brought up in the UK but whose parents came from the Caribbean.

Appearance and behaviour – You are well presented and somewhat overweight.

History
Freely divulged to doctor – You came to see the doctor 3 months ago after injuring your right ankle and a routine blood pressure check found that it was up a little. You were told to eat a healthier diet and try and lose some weight and to come back and have your blood pressure re-checked in a month's time. When you returned 6 weeks later your ankle was better but your blood pressure was still up and the doctor arranged some blood tests and a urine test. You also had a long discussion about changes you could make to your diet and lifestyle to try to get your blood pressure down. You saw the nurse today who checked your blood pressure again and asked you to wait to see the doctor. You feel 'a bit of a fraud' as you feel so well.

Divulged to doctor if specifically asked – Over the last 3 months you have tried to lose weight and eat a healthier diet but it has been difficult. You know that you are overweight but this does not really bother you. You think of yourself as fairly fit for your age. You still play football with your sons and friends in the park on Sundays. You have never had any chest pains, shortness of breath, palpitations, headaches or any other symptoms that have worried you. You drink five or six cups of coffee most days.

Ideas, concerns and expectations – Although today you are seeing the third different GP about your blood pressure, you are not bothered by this – both the previous doctors seemed very thorough – and you understand that it is not always possible to see the same doctor. You are a little confused about why everyone seems so interested in your blood pressure, when you feel absolutely fine and have not had any symptoms. Last time the doctor mentioned that you may need to take tablets for the rest of your life, which bothers you as you have always thought of yourself as a healthy individual and not someone who takes tablets. You were not sure what all the blood tests were for and you are a little worried that there may be something else that the doctors have not mentioned, to warrant all the tests. Last month your partner bought you a home blood pressure machine so you could check your blood pressure at home. You bought a relaxation tape as you thought this might help your blood pressure and you want to ask the doctor about this.

First words spoken to doctor – "The nurse said to see you to get the results of my blood tests and have a chat about my blood pressure."

Past medical history – You rarely come to see the doctor. When you were with your previous GP surgery, you suffered from gout in your left big toe on two occasions 4 years ago but have been fine since. You sprained your right ankle playing football 3 months ago and only booked to come to see the GP at your partner's insistence as she thought you might have broken something. The ankle problem cleared up with anti-inflammatory painkillers.

Drug history – You were prescribed medication to help prevent further gout attacks when you were registered at your previous practice, but you decided not to take these. You do not take any regular medication. You are not allergic to any drugs.

Social history – You live with your partner and two adult sons in a semi-detached house. You have run your own business – selling kitchen units – for 30 years. You drive a small van for work. You smoked 20 cigarettes a day from when you were 15 years old until 10 years ago when you stopped because you were getting short of breath playing football. You know that you drink a little too much – you often have four pints of lager on Friday and Saturday nights in the local pub, and one or two cans of lager most week nights at home after work.

Family history – Your father died of a heart attack when he was 72. Your mother had high blood pressure in her 70s but did not need any tablets for it. She died of breast cancer aged 76. Your older brother has had high blood pressure for the last 5 years. He is now 65 years old. He takes a couple of tablets every day but is otherwise well.

- Having read the information given to the simulated patient, what do you now think this station is testing?
- Make notes or discuss your thoughts with a colleague before you turn the page.

Review your approach to this station:

Tested at this station:

1. Data gathering
2. Data interpretation
3. Explanation of diagnosis
4. Management of common medical conditions presenting in primary care

Domain 2 – Data gathering, examination and clinical assessment skills

Data gathering

This patient has been found to have raised blood pressure (BP) on a number of occasions. Data gathering at this station should include appropriate history taking and review of his various BP readings:

- History:
  - Does he smoke?
  - Any family history of heart attacks, heart problems, high blood pressure or strokes?
  - Any chest pain, palpitations or shortness of breath?
  - Does he ever wake up at night gasping for breath? How many pillows does he use at night? Do his ankles swell up?
  - Any problems with pains in his legs when he walks?
  - Any headaches?
  - You already know that he is not diabetic from the blood glucose result.
  - Any family history of high cholesterol?
  - Any other medical problems in the past?
  - Does he take any medication?
- Review of BP readings – he has had three BP readings at the surgery over the last 3 months which have all been > 140/90, although none has been > 160/100.

Data interpretation

You have the results of the patient's recent blood tests and his BP readings. You also have access to cardiovascular risk prediction charts (also found in the back of the BNF). You need to be able to demonstrate that you can interpret these data in light of current best practice guidelines to help inform management options:

- Given his age, raised BP and raised cholesterol, you should calculate his cardiovascular disease (CVD) risk to see whether he needs to be on appropriate treatment.
- CVD risk is defined as non-fatal myocardial infarction (MI) and stroke, coronary and stroke death and new angina pectoris.
- When deciding whether to use the 'Non-smoker' or 'Smoker' risk prediction charts, it is recommended that you assess those who have given up smoking within 5 years using the 'Smoker' charts. This patient gave up 10 years ago, so is appropriately assessed using the 'Non-smoker' charts.

- CVD risk is underestimated by the charts for those with a family history of premature CVD – namely, first-degree female relative aged < 65 years or male < 55 years. This patient's father was 72 years old when he had his heart attack and so there is no need to apply the 1.5 risk multiplier recommended for those with a family history of premature CVD.
- Select the appropriate risk prediction chart – namely 'Non-diabetic men' and 'Non-smoker' and 'Age 50–59'.
- From the blood test results you know that the total cholesterol (TC) to HDL ratio is 6.0:1.0 = 6. If you plot where the x axis for TC to HDL of 6 intersects with a systolic BP of 156 you can see that this is clearly within the CVD risk > 20% over the next 10 years.
- Hence this patient is at significant CVD risk.
- The risk prediction charts may underestimate CVD risk in some ethnic minorities. In patients from the Indian sub-continent it is recommended to multiply the calculated risk by 1.5 to obtain a more realistic value. This patient is Black British with parents from the Caribbean. There are tools such as the ETHRISK calculator which adjusts the CVD risk for certain ethnic groups by re-calibrating the Framingham risk equations (see Further reading).

Domain I – Interpersonal skills

Explanation of diagnosis

Explaining to patients what you think is wrong with them in terms they can readily understand and which incorporate their own health beliefs is a key communication skill:

- You are the fourth health professional this patient has seen about his BP. You could enquire whether he has any concerns about this. What did the other doctors and nurse explain about high BP?
- What are his own health beliefs about BP? Are any family members or friends having treatment for BP? Has he discussed the matter with them?
- Does he know why we are interested in raised blood pressure, even when someone does not have any symptoms? You need to explain our understanding that over time high BP can damage blood vessels and put a strain on the heart.
- Does he understand why the other doctor ordered the blood tests? You could explain how the blood tests look at different things – whether there is any problem with his kidneys, whether he has diabetes and if his cholesterol is raised.
- Communicating risk – using the charts you can explain how we calculate the patient's risk of developing CVD. If someone scores ≥ 20% – in other words a 2 out of 10 chance or more – of developing CVD in the next 10 years then you can explain that we usually advise starting medication.
- You can explain that treatment may include drugs to lower blood pressure, aspirin to reduce the risk of blood clots (only when the BP is controlled to < 150/90) and a statin drug to lower cholesterol. Lifestyle factors such as diet and exercise are also very important (see below).
- You can use the risk assessment process to aid discussion with the patient and potentially encourage concordance.

- It is worth asking how the patient feels about having high BP. His self-image as a fit, healthy individual was challenged by the previous doctor's mention of having to take medication long term.
- This patient wants advice on relaxation tapes and home BP monitoring. He is already starting to take responsibility for his own BP management and you should positively reinforce this behaviour. You could advise him to bring his home BP machine to the surgery for the nurse to check the calibration and to get advice on how to self-monitor his BP. You can tell him that relaxation techniques may lead to modest reductions in BP.

Domain 3 – Clinical management skills

Management of common medical conditions presenting in primary care

Management of the risk factors for cardiovascular problems is a key aspect of health promotion activity in primary care. Hypertension is one modifiable risk factor that all GPs should feel confident in treating:

- Lifestyle advice is a key element in controlling BP, whether or not patients require antihypertensive medication. You should positively reinforce the fact that he has given up smoking and is physically active, and discuss how he has tried to address his alcohol intake and weight. Dietary advice to help reduce BP should include cutting down on salt and discouraging excessive caffeine consumption.
- This patient has tried making lifestyle changes to help lower his BP over the last 3 months, with little success. He currently meets the threshold to be offered drug therapy for his hypertension. According to NICE guidelines, calcium channel blockers or thiazide diuretics would be first-line options given his profile (see Knowledge-base). However, this patient has suffered from gout in the past which makes a thiazide diuretic less suitable.
- If you are going to write a prescription for him today, you might consider starting amlodipine 5 mg OD. Remember to discuss side effects with him, such as abdominal pain, nausea, palpitations and swollen ankles. Is he happy to take this medication?
- What does he think about cholesterol lowering tablets? Does he understand how these can help reduce his CVD risk? Would he be happy to give one a try? Simvastatin 20 mg nocte would be one option. Again, advise him of side effects such as upset stomach, rash, hypersensitivity, headache and muscle aches.
- You should also explain that aspirin 75 mg OD reduces the risk of cardiovascular events by reducing the chance of clots forming in blood vessels. However, he should not start this until his BP is controlled to < 150/90.
- Do not forget to check allergy status before prescribing any drugs – this patient has no known allergies.
- He did not take his gout prophylaxis medication previously, when prescribed. You need to understand his reasons for this as his past behaviour may be relevant to future concordance.
- The GP curriculum notes that many patients do not take their preventative cardiovascular medication and that you need to respect patient autonomy when reaching a management plan. Is he really planning to take his new medication and does he have any further questions about the tablets?

- He has not had an ECG. This would be helpful in looking for left ventricular strain. Explain what this test involves and address any questions he may have.
- It would be prudent to check his urate levels, given his history of gout.
- Ask him to see you again in 1 month for a review, or sooner if he has any concerns.

Knowledge-base – Management of hypertension

References – NICE guidelines 2006, BNF, DVLA 2007.

Hypertension	<ul><li>Persistent raised BP > 140/90</li><li>Raised BP on two subsequent clinic visits following initial raised BP</li><li>BP should be assessed from two readings on each visit under the best conditions</li></ul>
Lifestyle advice	Offer lifestyle advice initially and then periodically for those being assessed or treated for hypertension
Antihypertensive drug therapy	Offer drug therapy if persistently raised BP:<ul><li>≥ 160/100</li><li>>140/90 and existing CVD or CVD risk ≥ 20% over 10 years or target organ damage</li></ul>
Treatment targets	<ul><li>Aim of treatment is to reduce BP to 140/90 or below</li><li>Patients often require more than one drug to achieve this target</li></ul>
Other drugs	<ul><li>Aspirin – used for primary prevention to reduce CVD risk in those aged over 50 who have CVD risk ≥ 20% over 10 years. Unduly high BP must be controlled first</li><li>Statins – used for primary prevention to reduce CVD risk in those aged over 40 with raised BP who have CVD risk ≥ 20% over 10 years</li></ul>
Elderly patients	Offer the same treatment to patients over 80 years old as you would to those aged over 55, bearing in mind co-morbidity and drug interactions
Secondary causes of raised BP	<ul><li>Kidney disease (e.g. renal artery stenosis)</li><li>Cushing's syndrome</li><li>Conn's syndrome</li><li>Hyperparathyroidism</li><li>Acromegaly</li><li>Phaeochromocytoma</li><li>Coarctation of aorta</li></ul>Specialist referral is required if you suspect a secondary cause or if the patient has signs of accelerated (malignant) hypertension
DVLA	<ul><li>Group 1 drivers – can continue driving and not required to inform DVLA unless treatment causes unacceptable side effects</li><li>Group 2 drivers – stop driving and notify DVLA if systolic ≥ 180 or diastolic ≥ 100</li></ul>
Continuing care	<ul><li>Annual review with patients to monitor BP, discuss lifestyle, provide support, assess medication use and side effects</li></ul>

NICE 2006. Choosing drugs for patients newly diagnosed with hypertension. In: Hypertension: management of hypertension in adults in primary care (Quick Reference Guide). London: NICE. www.nice.org.uk. Reproduced with permission.

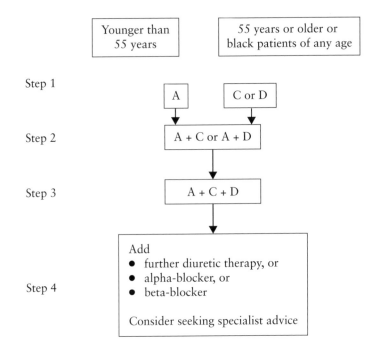

A = ACE inhibitor (consider angiotensin-II receptor antagonist if ACE intolerant)
C = calcium channel blocker
D = thiazide diuretic
Black patients are those of African or Caribbean descent, and not mixed-race, Asian or Chinese patients

Take home messages

- Data interpretation is a key skill that can be assessed in the CSA.
- Explain diagnoses to patients in terms they can understand.
- Lifestyle advice is a fundamental element in the management of hypertension.

Ideas for further revision

Explaining new diagnoses to patients is a common occurrence in primary care. Practise trying to explain diagnoses such as osteoarthritis, COPD, asthma, diabetes and thyroid disease in simple, accurate, jargon-free terms.

Further reading

British National Formulary (BNF). Published jointly by BMJ Publishing Group and RPS Publishing, London. Updated every 6 months. www.bnf.org.

British Hypertension Society. www.bhsoc.org/default.stm.

Drivers and Vehicles Licensing Agency. *For Medical Practitioners: At a Glance Guide to the Current Medical Standards of Fitness to Drive.* Swansea: DVLA, February 2007. www.dvla.gov.uk/medical/ataglance.aspx.

ETHRISK – A modified Framingham CHD and CVD risk calculator for British Black and minority ethnic groups. www.epi.bris.ac.uk/CVDethrisk.

Joint British Societies' Guidelines on the Prevention of Cardiovascular Disease in Clinical Practice: Risk Assessment. British Heart Foundation Factfile. January 2006. www.bhsoc.org/bhf_factfiles/bhf_factfile_jan_2006.pdf.

NICE guidelines – Hypertension: management of hypertension in adults in primary care. Clinical guidelines 34 (partial update of NICE clinical guidelines 18) June 2006. www.nice.org.uk/CG034.

RCGP curriculum statement 15.1 – Clinical Management: Cardiovascular problems. www.rcgp.org.uk.

Information given to candidates

Mavis O'Brien is a 74-year-old patient and mother of one of the practice nurses.

Her past medical history includes a myocardial infarction (MI) 10 years ago. She has not had angina pains since the MI.

She is prescribed the following medication:

Aspirin   75 mg OD
Atenolol   50 mg OD
Ramipril   2.5 mg OD
Simvastatin   20 mg nocte

At the last consultation 6 months ago, the patient was very upset over the death of Edna, her best friend.

The first thing the patient says as she enters the consultation rooms is, "I've been getting ever so dizzy doctor over the last few months. I wonder if it's to do with my nerves. I want you to sort me out."

- What do you think this station is testing?
- Make notes or discuss your thoughts with a colleague before you read on.

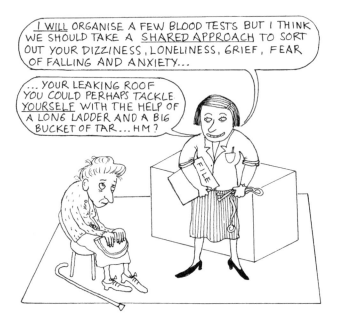

Plan your approach to this station:

Information given to simulated patient

Basic details – You are Mavis O'Brien, a Caucasian 74-year-old retired school-teacher and widow.

Appearance and behaviour – You are anxious and fidgety, and talk rather fast. But if you feel the doctor is kind and understanding then you will begin to relax a little and slow down. During the consultation you repeatedly ask the doctor if he or she can 'sort things out' for you.

History

Freely divulged to doctor – You started having dizzy spells 5 or 6 months ago. They can last from a few seconds to several minutes. Your daughter thought that you should come to see the doctor as she is worried about your symptoms, although you have never blacked out or fallen during these episodes. You miss your friend and companion Edna terribly, since she died 6 months ago, and you think that the dizziness may be due to her death affecting your 'nerves'.

Divulged to doctor if specifically asked – You find it hard to describe exactly what the dizziness feels like. The best description you can give is that you feel a little lightheaded. Sometimes you get several episodes of dizziness in one day, then nothing for over a week. There does not seem to be any pattern to when they come on – for instance, you have not noticed things being worse after you stand up, or if you move your head suddenly. You do seem to get more anxious these days and when you are dizzy you sometimes notice that you are breathing faster. Your ears have been fine. You have not experienced any chest pain, palpitations, weakness or odd sensations in your limbs. You do not feel sick or particularly unsteady on your feet when the dizziness comes on. You have not noticed any problem with your eyesight. You have not felt depressed or down, just somewhat lonely.

Ideas, concerns and expectations – You think that the dizziness may just be your 'nerves' as you have not been yourself since your good friend Edna died 6 months ago. You miss her and feel more anxious about your own health, and have started to think more and more about your own mortality. You are also concerned that you might fall and that you are on your own. You want the doctor to sort you out and solve all these problems for you. But if you feel confident in the doctor and they explain that it is unlikely to be anything serious and probably, as you suspect, down to your nerves, you will be able to accept this. You feel that you take enough tablets as it is, and do not want to take any more. But you are happy to have some blood tests and see the doctor again.

First words spoken to doctor – "I've been getting ever so dizzy doctor over the last few months. I wonder if it's to do with my nerves. I want you to sort me out."

Past medical history – You had a heart attack 10 years ago from which you made a good recovery. You also suffer from osteoarthritis in your hips and knees.

Drug history – You take various tablets following your heart attack, including aspirin 75 mg once a day ('to help thin the blood'), atenolol 50 mg once a day ('to help the heart'), ramipril 2.5 mg once a day (you are not sure why you take this) and simvastatin 20 mg at night ('to help the cholesterol'). You take an occasional paracetamol for pains in your hips and knees.

Social history – You have lived on your own since your husband died 15 years ago and have never required any home help, other than your daughter who visits several times a week and takes you shopping. Since your friend died you go out much less frequently. You used to do everything together – bingo, dancing, lunch clubs and bowls, but it just does not seem the same going on your own, and you worry about falling with the dizzy spells. You smoked 20 cigarettes a day for over 30 years, but stopped about 10 years before your heart attack. You have the odd glass of sherry on special occasions. You do not drive.

Family history – There are no major medical problems in your immediate family.

- Having read the information given to the simulated patient, what do you now think this station is testing?
- Make notes or discuss your thoughts with a colleague before you turn the page.

Review your approach to this station:

Tested at this station:

1. Encouraging patients to take responsibility for their health and well-being
2. History taking skills
3. Physical examination
4. Managing uncertainty

Domain I – Interpersonal skills

Encouraging patients to take responsibility for their health and well-being (overlap with Domain 3)

Patients often present to their GP surgery expecting the doctor to 'fix' whatever problems they have, whether they are medically related or not. Encouraging patients to take some responsibility and to adopt self-help measures, where appropriate and with support, is a key skill that you should be able to demonstrate:

- This patient has a number of problems – loneliness, grief, anxiety, worries about falling and being on her own, and dizziness. She will try and place the responsibility for dealing with these problems on you, and expects you to provide solutions.
- Although you may be able to help, it is important to explain to the patient that there is much that she can do to address these issues herself (see Managing uncertainty).
- One response to the patient's opening statement might be – *"Well let's discuss this further and see what we can both do to try and improve things."* This signals that she too will need to take on some responsibility.
- In this case you may feel under particular pressure to 'solve' the patient's various problems, as her daughter is one of your colleagues at the practice. But by encouraging the patient to tackle some of these issues herself, you can empower her to be an active agent in her own health promotion.

Domain 2 – Data gathering, examination and clinical assessment skills

History taking skills

You need to take a focused history to try and identify the cause of her dizziness. But remember that you will score more marks and obtain key details if you start with open questions and elicit the patient's ideas, concerns and expectations before moving on to more specific, closed questions:

- She is getting dizzy and thinks this may be due to her 'nerves' – can she say more about this?
- What are her thoughts about what is going on?
- Does she have any particular concerns about these symptoms?
- What was she hoping would happen from coming to see the doctor today?
- 'Dizziness' is an imprecise term that needs to be clarified. Does she mean that she feels faint at certain times or is she describing a sensation of movement – e.g. spinning – when there is none?

- What is she doing when she gets these dizzy spells? Has she just stood up or moved her head?
- Any problems with her ears? Any ringing or deafness?
- Does she vomit or feel nauseous when she feels dizzy?
- Any palpitations or chest pain?
- Any similar symptoms to when she had her heart attack?
- Does she smoke?
- She mentions her 'nerves'. What has her mood been like recently – has she felt low? Do any situations make her feel anxious?
- Does she find herself breathing faster when the dizziness comes on? Does she feel anxious first and then dizzy?
- Has she fallen or banged her head recently?
- Has she blacked out or lost consciousness?
- Any weakness or numbness in her arms or legs? Any visual problems?
- Is her neck stiff or sore?
- Has she had a cough recently or pain passing urine? Has she been feverish?
- Does she drive?

Physical examination

Although there is a lot to cover at this station, do not neglect to examine the patient. You will be expected to examine her ears (see Examination 1: Station 6) and perform a brief cardiovascular examination (see below). You will subsequently be told that there are no abnormal findings. If you indicate that you wish to perform further examinations, such as a full neurological examination, neck movements, or Hallpike test (positional manoeuvre to induce vertigo), then you will be informed that this is not necessary and to assume that the findings are normal.

- The patient is complaining of dizziness and has a history of cardiovascular disease.
- As part of a brief cardiovascular examination you would be expected to examine her:
  - Pulse
  - BP, including checking for a postural drop
  - Carotids for any bruits
  - Heart sounds at the four standard precordium sites: mitral, tricuspid, pulmonary and aortic areas.
- You may be tempted to perform a more thorough cardiovascular examination (see Further reading); however, there is limited time for the consultation and what is expected is a focused examination.

Domain 3 – Clinical management skills

Managing uncertainty

One of the specific problem-solving competencies, as set out in the new GP curriculum, is the ability to manage conditions that may present in an undifferentiated way. You are expected to be able to demonstrate when you can reassure patients, when expectant management is appropriate ('watchful waiting') and when you need to initiate diagnostic tests or treatment – taking into account the patient's wishes. In this case, the cause of the patient's dizziness is not completely clear from the history and examination findings today:

- This is a deliberately complex and challenging station. The patient presents with several issues: the feelings of loss for her friend, increasing anxiety over her own health, and episodes of lightheadedness with no clear diagnostic pattern. Additionally, she wants you to take responsibility for her problems and to solve them for her.
- In a 10 min consultation you need to be able to elicit her own agenda, take a focused history and examination to try and help diagnose the cause of her dizziness, and offer her management options that are acceptable both to you and to her. You also need to try and get her to take on some responsibility for her problems.
- This is unlikely to be a one-off consultation with the patient and you need to think about what would be most appropriate – and safe – to do at this first meeting.
- You might be tempted to send her for a range of investigations, including blood tests, 24 h BP monitoring, 24 h ECG recording, tilt test, MRI scan of her head and neck X-rays, or even to refer her to an elderly care specialist today. However, if you suspect that her symptoms are related to anxiety and grief, then a more appropriate way forward may be to make providing support and advice your main priority, together with incremental investigations.
- You can reassure the patient that there are no worrying findings on examination. Explain that you are unsure of the exact diagnosis, although – as she suggests – the dizziness may be related to her anxieties and grief at the loss of her friend.
- Given the uncertainty about the diagnosis, her age, and past medical history, you would be expected to organize some preliminary blood tests – e.g. FBC, U&Es, glucose, LFTs and TFTs – and arrange to review her with the results. Is she happy with this plan?
- Various self-help management options which you could suggest include:
  - Having her eyes tested at the optician.
  - Attending a local bereavement group or bereavement counselling.
  - Has she thought about a pendant alarm to wear to allay her anxieties about falling at home?
  - Would she feel safer and enjoy the company provided by sheltered accommodation?
  - How does she feel about trying to go along to the groups she used to attend, or accessing befriending/buddy support services through organizations such as Age Concern or Help the Aged?
  - Could she ask her daughter to take her out more?
- You could also offer a trial of a vestibular sedative such as cinnarize 15 mg TDS. However, she is not keen to take any more medication and you should respect this.
- Safety netting – make sure the patient knows what to do if she develops any new symptoms, such as chest pain or blackouts.

- The key to managing uncertainty is to ensure that whatever plan is agreed, it is acceptable to both doctor and patient. Is she happy with the advice about sources of help, that you are doing some basic tests, and that you will review things in 2 weeks, or sooner if required?

Knowledge-base – Dizziness

References – RCGP curriculum statement 15.7, Colledge et al. (1996) – see Further reading.

Causes

Neurological	<ul><li>Stroke:<ul><li>○ Brainstem or cerebellar</li><li>○ Haemorrhage or infarction</li></ul></li><li>Trauma and concussion</li><li>Peripheral neuropathy</li><li>Multiple sclerosis</li><li>Parkinsonism</li><li>Brain tumours</li><li>Multisystem atrophy</li><li>Vestibular aura of migraine</li></ul>
Otological	<ul><li>Peripheral:<ul><li>○ Labyrinthitis</li><li>○ Ménière's disease (vertigo, tinnitus, deafness)</li><li>○ Benign paroxysmal vertigo (BPV)</li><li>○ Ramsay Hunt syndrome</li></ul></li><li>Central:<ul><li>○ Acoustic neuroma</li></ul></li></ul>
Cardiovascular	<ul><li>Arrhythmias</li><li>Postural hypotension</li></ul>
Psychological	<ul><li>Anxiety</li><li>Hyperventilation</li></ul>
Drugs	<ul><li>Antihypertensives</li><li>Vasodilators</li><li>Antidepressants</li><li>Parkinson's disease medication (e.g. levodopa, selegiline)</li><li>Phosphodiesterase-5 inhibitors (e.g. sildenafil)</li></ul>
Other	<ul><li>Poor vision</li><li>Cervical spondylosis</li><li>Osteoarthritis</li><li>Hypoglycaemia</li></ul>

Management in elderly patients

Chronic dizziness in an elderly patient

History
Character – Vertigo, light headedness, or unsteadiness
Provocative factors – For e.g., postural change, head or neck movement, anxiety, none (occurs spontaneously)
Associated symptoms – Blackouts, falls, tinnitus, or hearing loss

Test visual acuity
Assess anxiety
Take smoking history

Are there blackouts? → Yes → Refer for 24 hour electrocardiography and carotid sinus massage

No

Is there vertigo with tinnitus and hearing loss? → Yes → Refer to otolaryngologist

No

Are there symptoms/abnormalities during:

- Vigorous head and neck movement? → Yes → • Cervical spondylosis
- Measurement of blood pressure while erect and supine? → Yes → • Postural hypotension
- Heel to toe walking (if abnormal examine neuromotor system in legs?) → Yes → • Cerebrovascular disease
- Two minutes of voluntary overbreathing? → Yes → • Hyperventilation
- Hallpike manoeuvre (see text for details)? → Yes → • Benign positional vertigo

Is dizziness associated with falls? → Yes → Refer to geriatrician

Do findings fit diagnostic criteria? → No → Refer to geriatrician

From Colledge et al (1996). Reproduced with permission from BMJ Publishing Group.

Take home messages

- In general practice conditions often present in an undifferentiated way. You need to be comfortable dealing with diagnostic uncertainty.
- Encourage patients to take responsibility for their health and well-being, with appropriate support and advice.
- Physical examinations needs to be slick and focused given the limited time at each CSA station.

Ideas for further revision

The simulated patients in the CSA will be similar to those you encounter in an ordinary GP surgery; so you would be wise to ensure that for each of the common presenting conditions – dizziness, back pain, headaches, indigestion, irregular periods, pill requests, abdominal pain, etc. – you have a mental check list for history taking, examination and management options.

Further reading

Colledge NR, Barr-Hamilton RM, Lewis SJ, Sellar RJ, Wilson JA. Evaluation of investigations to diagnose the cause of dizziness in elderly people: a community based controlled study. *BMJ* 1996;**313**:788–792. www.bmj.com.

Department of Health. *The National Service Framework for Older People*. London: Department of Health, 2001. www.dh.gov.uk/en/ Publicationsandstatistics/Publications/PublicationsPolicyAndGuidance/ DH_4003066.

NHS National Library for Health Clinical Knowledge Summaries – Vertigo. www.cks.library.nhs.uk/clinical_knowledge.

RCGP curriculum statement 15.7 – Clinical Management: Neurological Problems. www.rcgp.org.uk.

Thomas J, Monaghan T. *Oxford Handbook of Clinical Examination and Practical Skills*. Oxford: Oxford University Press, 2007.

Information given to candidates

Zoë Brighthouse is a 16-year-old patient whose parents and older sister are also registered with the practice.

Her records show that she attended the surgery a week ago with her mother and saw one of the Foundation Year 2 doctors.

At that time she was complaining of a week's history of sore throat and general malaise.

Examination is documented as:

Chest	Clear
Otoscopy	Normal
Throat	?Exudate on tonsils
Neck	Enlarged lymph nodes anterior cervical chain

She was prescribed amoxicillin 500 mg TDS for ?tonsillitis.

She had been prescribed amoxicillin for an ear infection earlier in the year without any problems.

The patient is on her own today.

As the patient enters the room she says, "I've stopped those tablets the other doctor gave me because they made me come out in a rash."

- What do you think this station is testing?
- Make notes or discuss your thoughts with a colleague before you read on.

Plan your approach to this station:

Information given to simulated patient

Basic details – You are Zoë Brighthouse, a Caucasian 16-year-old pupil at the local state school.

Appearance and behaviour – You are quiet and take a while to open up to the doctor. But if you feel that the doctor has a caring and understanding manner, then you are more likely to be forthcoming earlier in the consultation about your true concerns about HIV (see Ideas, concerns and expectations).

History

Freely divulged to doctor – You have been feeling 'awful' for a couple of weeks now with a sore throat, fever, general aches and pains, and tiredness. Last week you saw one of the other doctors at the practice with your mother and you were prescribed antibiotics for a throat infection. The same day you started the tablets you came out in a fine red rash all over your body, so you have not taken any more. The rash has now settled. You were not able to book an earlier appointment than today.

Divulged to doctor if specifically asked – You have only missed 3 days off school in the last 2 weeks. You have not had a cough or brought up any phlegm. You have not vomited and you have not suffered from diarrhoea or constipation. You have not had any abdominal pain or pain passing urine. You are not going to the toilet to urinate more frequently and you do not have excessive thirst. Two weeks ago you had vaginal sex with a boy from your class who you do not know very well, after a party at the home of a friend. You did not have oral sex. It was the first time you had ever had sex. You asked him to use a condom – which he did – as you are not on the pill and were worried about getting pregnant. You do not think there were any problems such as the condom splitting. You only had a couple of drinks that night and felt in control of the situation. The sex was consensual. You have not had any genital symptoms, such as itchiness or a discharge. You have never had any genital infections. You did a pregnancy test last week 'just to make sure', which was negative. Your periods are always regular and you started your period on time 4 days ago. You did not tell the doctor last week about having had sex as your mother was with you.

Ideas, concerns and expectations – You are upset with yourself as you had planned not to have sex until you were older, with someone you loved. You think that the tablets probably did cause the rash but read on the internet that when you are infected with HIV you can develop an illness with general aches and pains, a sore throat and a rash – just like your symptoms. Even though you used a condom when you had sex, you are still worried that you could have got a sexually transmitted infection, such as HIV. You have heard of condoms splitting without people knowing and this has been preying on your mind. You have never wanted to take the oral contraceptive pill or any hormonal alternatives as you 'don't want to put all those hormones in your body.' You want advice from the doctor on the chances of you having HIV and whether you should have an HIV test.

First words spoken to doctor – "I've stopped those tablets the other doctor gave me because they made me come out in a rash."

Past medical history – You had eczema as a child but are no longer affected by this. You rarely go to see the doctor as you are generally fit and well. You had an ear infection earlier this year which settled with antibiotics.

Drug history – You do not take any regular medication and only took one of the antibiotic tablets the doctor prescribed last week. You took the antibiotic amoxicillin for an ear infection early this year without any problems. As far as you know you are not allergic to any medication. You do not use any illicit drugs.

Social history – You live with your parents and sister who is 1 year older than you. You are doing well at school and have GCSE exams coming up at the end of this academic year. You are popular at school and have a close group of friends. You have the odd cigarette when you are out but you do not really like smoking. You are sensible about drinking alcohol – you never get really drunk – but you do drink several alcopops when you go out with your friends at the weekend.

Family history – There are no major health problems in your family.

- Having read the information given to the simulated patient, what do you now think this station is testing?
- Make notes or discuss your thoughts with a colleague before you turn the page.

Review your approach to this station:

Tested at this station:

1. Identifying a hidden agenda
2. History taking from a reticent patient
3. Reaching a shared management plan with an adolescent

Domain 1 – Interpersonal skills

Identifying a hidden agenda

Patients often present with a problem that is not the main reason for their attendance at the surgery. You need to be open to the possibility of such hidden agendas and allow the patient every opportunity to disclose their true concerns:

- It can be daunting for a teenager to see a doctor on their own. To create the right environment for her to open up you need to employ excellent communication skills through active listening, showing empathy and encouraging her to contribute as an equal partner in the consultation.
- Your attitude to anything she tells you about her health or health concerns must be non-judgemental and supportive. Patients often test you out early on in the consultation to see if you are the sort of doctor they feel happy to disclose more personal information to.
- Pick up on any clues that the patient may give – e.g. *"You seem very anxious about what has happened – do you think there might be something else going on other than a throat infection?"*
- Stay patient-focused and if you feel there is a mismatch between your worries about the presenting complaint and the patient's, then explore her ideas, concerns and expectations further.

Domain 2 – Data gathering, examination and clinical assessment skills

History taking from a reticent patient

There is the potential for this scenario to be challenging in terms of time management, as the patient is initially slow in giving a history. But if she feels that you have a caring and understanding manner, then she is more likely to offer the information you need to safely manage the consultation while also addressing her agenda:

- You could ask whether the patient came with anyone today – e.g. she may have a friend in the waiting room. If so, would she like them to come in to give her some support?
- If during the consultation you suspect that she may want to disclose further information, but seems reluctant, remind her that your discussion is confidential.
- Ask her to recap on what has happened over the last couple of weeks, as this allows you to find out her understanding of events, including last week's visit to see your colleague.

- Ask about any allergies to medication. Check that when she was prescribed amoxicillin earlier in the year for an ear infection she did not have any similar reaction.
- The clear history from the notes, together with the information about a rash starting soon after taking the antibiotics, should alert you early on to the probable diagnosis of infectious mononucleosis (glandular fever).
- However, be careful not to close down the consultation early, and ensure that you still ask questions about her health beliefs, concerns and expectations, or you will miss the key element to this scenario – namely, the patient's anxiety about possible HIV infection.
- Allow the patient time to discuss her concerns regarding having had sex and her worries about HIV infection.
- You should take a full sexual history (see Examination 1: Station 5) to assess HIV risk.
- Use words that the patient can understand – do not assume that what you might consider simple terms are readily understood, e.g. 'vagina'.
- Given her age it is also important to find out if the sex was consensual. Enquire about the age of her sexual partner – if he was significantly older, then you might be worried that there was an element of coercion.
- Ask about her mood – has she felt low or depressed? How are things at school? How is life at home?
- Has she been able to discuss her worries with anyone else – either friends or family?

Physical examination

If you say that you would like to examine the patient, you will be told that this is not necessary and to assume that the findings are the same as when she was seen last week (see Information given to candidates).

Domain 3 – Clinical management skills

Reaching a shared management plan with an adolescent (overlap with Domain 1)

In addition to reassuring the patient over her main concern – the risk of HIV infection – this consultation is also an opportunity to cover wider health promotion issues:

- You should explain how the history suggests a diagnosis of glandular fever, although she would need a blood test to confirm this. You can reassure her that this is a common condition, caused by a virus (Epstein–Barr) and is usually a short self-limiting illness – although it can run a protracted course in some cases. You can explain how it is spread – by saliva – and therefore that she should avoid kissing and sharing cups and towels while she is still unwell.
- Advise rest, plenty of fluids and simple painkillers – such as paracetamol and ibuprofen – together with self-help measures such as gargling with salt water for her sore throat.
- Is she happy to have some blood taken to confirm the diagnosis (FBC to look for leukocytosis and monospot)?

- Reassure her that as she has just had her period and the pregnancy test was negative, she can feel confident that she is not pregnant.
- Reassure her that her risk of HIV would be assessed as low, as she had protected sex, and there would therefore be little indication for having an HIV test. What does she think about this?
- If, despite your reassurances, she feels that for piece of mind she would still like to have the test, then you should advise her to wait 3 months after having had sex – the 'window period' – as the test detects antibodies to the virus and the body takes time to produce these. In the interim she should use condoms.
- Be positive about her proven ability to negotiate practising safer sex – using a condom – and encourage continued use. Advise her where she can get these herself rather than having to rely on a partner. Often there are local resources such as a Young People's Project, Teenage Health Bus, or schemes such as C-card where teenagers can show a card at Genitourinary Medicine (GUM) or Family Planning clinics to get free condoms, without the embarrassment of having to ask a receptionist or pharmacist.
- Has she considered other forms of contraception?
- Offer information on sexual health screening services at GUM clinics or at the surgery – e.g. swabs or a urine sample to screen for infections such as chlamydia. Does she know anything about these sorts of services?
- The GP curriculum states that every consultation with a child or young person should be an opportunity for general health promotion advice. How much exercise does she do? What is her diet like? Does she use alcohol or illicit drugs? Are there any small steps she could realistically take to make her lifestyle healthier?
- Encourage her to discuss what has happened with her parents or sister. If she does not feel comfortable speaking to her family, is there any other adult she could talk to, such as a teacher, school nurse or youth worker who she trusts?
- Remember to negotiate all the above with the patient, rather than simply telling her what steps she can take.
- Check her understanding at regular intervals during the consultation and ask her to explain the plan you have jointly agreed back to you.

Knowledge-base – Children, consent, confidentiality and the law

References – Department of Health guidance, House of Lords *Gillick* case, and Family Law Reform Act 1969 – see Further reading.

	English law
Under 16 years old	• The House of Lord's judgement in the *Gillick* case (see Further reading) ruled that the consent of a child under 16 can – in certain circumstances – have legal effect. This applies even if the parents disagree with the child over the proposed treatment • Lord Scarman held that a test of capacity be applied, which could determine whether the young person had 'sufficient understanding and intelligence to enable him or her to understand fully what is proposed' (*Gillick* judgement page 423) • This has become known as *Gillick*-competence • However, patients under 16 who are *Gillick*-competent should still be encouraged to involve their parents
16 and 17 years old	• Although all those aged under 18 are classed as minors, the Family Law Reform Act 1969 gives statutory recognition to the consent of 16 and 17 year olds to any 'surgical, medical or dental treatment', making it 'as effective as it would be if he were of full age' (sections 8(1) & 8(3)) • In other words – as the Department of Health guidelines make clear – those aged 16 and 17 are presumed to have the competence to give consent for themselves
≥ 18 years old	Treated as adults under the law – i.e. presumed to be competent
Emergencies	As with adults, if a patient under 18 is not competent, e.g. if they are unconscious, and it is an emergency situation such that it is unreasonable to wait, then you are legally entitled to treat without consent, acting in the best interests of the patient
Consent versus refusal	• As the law currently stands, minors – namely all those under 18 years of age – are legally entitled to *consent* to medical treatment (so long as they are *Gillick*-competent if under 16), yet they do not have an absolute right to *refuse* medical treatment. This is because anyone with parental responsibility can legally give consent on behalf of a minor • However, in practice, it would be highly unlikely for a doctor to proceed with an intervention in the face of a competent child's refusal, even if the consent of someone with parental responsibility did technically mean that there was legal consent. This situation would require further discussion and potential involvement of the courts
Confidentiality	• You must keep confidential any information a competent child asks you not to disclose, unless you believe doing so would put the child or others at risk of serious harm • You should encourage the patient to involve their family, unless this is not in their best interests • You should consult with a senior colleague and your defence organization before taking the significant step of breaking confidentiality
Fraser guidelines	In the *Gillick* judgement, Lord Fraser listed criteria that must be met to allow doctors lawfully to give contraceptive advice and treatment to children under 16 without parental involvement: • The young person understands the advice • The young person cannot be persuaded to involve their parents • The young person is likely to begin or continue having sex with or without contraceptive treatment • The young person's physical or mental health, or both, is likely to suffer unless they receive treatment • The young person's best interests require them to have contraceptive advice or treatment without parental consent

Take home messages

- The key skill when dealing with adolescents and young people is treating them as real partners in the consultation.
- Picking up on cues from the patient will help identify hidden agendas.
- Signposting patients to support services and other agencies is important within primary care.

Ideas for further revision

Although this station was not specifically about consent issues in children, you could easily be presented in the CSA with either an adolescent or parent of a child under 16 years of age who has requested contraception or an abortion. Make sure you feel happy about how you would deal with such a situation and that you are familiar with the law and national guidance in this area.

Further reading

Department of Health. *Seeking Consent: Working with Children*. London: DoH, 2001. www.dh.gov.uk/en/Publicationsandstatistics/Publications/Publications PolicyAndGuidance/DH_4007005.

Department of Health. *'You're Welcome' Quality Criteria – Making Health Services Young People Friendly*. London: DoH, 2007. www.dh.gov.uk/en/ Publicationsandstatistics/Publications/PublicationsPolicyAndGuidance/ DH_073586.

Gillick v West Norfolk and Wisbech Area Health Authority and another [1985] 3 All ER 402.

NHS National Library for Health Clinical Knowledge Summaries – glandular fever. www.cks.library.nhs.uk/clinical_knowledge.

NICE – Prevention of sexually transmitted infections and under 18 conceptions. Public health intervention guidance 3. Quick reference guide, February 2007. www.nice.org.uk/guidance/PHI3/quickrefguide/pdf/English/download. dspx.

RCGP curriculum statement 8 – Care of children and young people. www. rcgp.org.uk.

Royal College of General Practitioners and Royal College of Nursing. *Getting it Right for Teenagers in Your Practice*. London: RCGP, 2002. www.rcn.org. uk/members/downloads/getting_it_right.pdf.

The Terence Higgins Trust – the leading HIV and AIDS charity in the UK. www.tht.org.uk.

General Medical Council (GMC). 0–18 years: guidance for all doctors. 2007. www.gmc-uk.org.

Information given to candidates

Michelle McKinley is a 20-year-old shop assistant who recently registered with your surgery.

She saw the practice nurse for a new patient check and her records state:

- Smoker – 10 cigarettes a day
- Alcohol – approximately 8 units a week
- Exercise – minimal
- Urinalysis – normal
- Blood pressure – 122/76
- Height 1.52 m; weight 72 kg; BMI 31 kg/m^2
- Just moved to the area with husband
- No children
- Taking folic acid 400 µg OD as trying for a baby

The first words the patient says as she enters the room are, "We've been trying for a baby for 6 months now but nothing seems to be happening doctor."

- What do you think this station is testing?
- Make notes or discuss your thoughts with a colleague before you turn the page.

Plan your approach to this station:

Information given to simulated patient

Basic details – You are Michelle McKinley, a Caucasian 20-year-old shop assistant.

Appearance and behaviour – You are casually dressed and come across as a little anxious. You speak very matter-of-factly about sex and your efforts to get pregnant.

History

Freely divulged to doctor – You were married 6 months ago and have been trying for a baby since then. You were living with your parents-in-law until last month when you and your husband moved into a rented flat in the next-door town. You do not understand why you are not pregnant yet, as your friends seem to be able to fall pregnant as soon as they stop taking the pill. You thought you should see the doctor to find out if you needed some tests.

Divulged to doctor if specifically asked – It was difficult when you were living in a room at your parents-in-law to have the privacy to have sexual intercourse regularly, but you still managed to do so at least once a week. For the last couple of months you have been trying to have lots of sex in the 5-day period right in the middle between your periods, as your mum said this was the best time to get pregnant. But doing this is making both you and your husband rather stressed and feeling 'under pressure', such that sex has now become more of a chore. Your periods were always regular – every 28 days – before you started on the pill (back when you were 16 years old), and returned to this pattern within a couple of months of stopping the pill 6 months ago. You have never had heavy periods, or bleeding between periods. You do not have any vaginal discharge. You have never had any sexually transmitted infections (STIs) and only had two previous boyfriends with whom you had sex, before you met your husband. You are having penetrative vaginal sex (your husband is putting his penis into your vagina and ejaculating sperm). You do not have excessive facial hair. Your weight is steady.

Ideas, concerns and expectations – You thought that as soon as you stopped taking the pill you would get pregnant. You know that sometimes older women take a while to get pregnant, but at your age you do not understand why there seems to be a 'problem'. Your mum said it could be your 'hormones' and you should see the doctor. You think the 'problem' must be your fault, as your husband was able to get a previous girlfriend pregnant, although she had an abortion. You have a sketchy idea of what happens each month when your body produces an egg and how that fits in with you having a period, but you would feel 'stupid' if you asked about this. If the doctor comes across as kind and understanding and reassures you that there is nothing to worry about, you will be happy with the consultation. You will try and take on board any general health advice the doctor gives you to help increase the chance of you becoming pregnant.

First words spoken to doctor – "We've been trying for a baby for 6 months now but nothing seems to be happening doctor."

Past medical history – You know that you are a little overweight and should give up smoking, but otherwise you think of yourself as fairly healthy. You have never had any medical problems in the past, apart from the odd ear or throat infection. You have never had an abortion or miscarriage, or ever been pregnant.

Drug history – You have been taking 400 μg of folic acid once a day for 6 months. Before you were married you used Microgynon 30 – 'the combined pill' – for contraception, which you started when you were 16 years old. You are not allergic to any medication.

Social history – You live with your husband, who has just qualified as an electrician, in rented accommodation. You and your husband both smoke about 10 cigarettes a day. You drink about four cans of normal strength lager over a week. You left school when you were 16 years old with four GCSE qualifications. You work as an assistant in a high street clothes shop.

Family history – There is no history of major health problems or infertility in your family. As far as you know, no-one has polycystic ovaries or had an early menopause.

- Having read the information given to the simulated patient, what do you now think this station is testing?
- Make notes or discuss your thoughts with a colleague before you turn the page.

Review your approach to this station:

Tested at this station:

1. History taking skills
2. Offering reassurance
3. Health promotion around fertility issues

Domain 2 – Data gathering, examination and clinical assessment skills

History taking skills

Simply from the patient's opening words you may feel that there is nothing to worry about here. But it is important to understand the patient's perspective on events and why she has attended now. You also need to exclude symptoms that would prompt investigation even at this early stage. Questions you could ask include:

● Why is she concerned about not being pregnant yet?
● What are her expectations of how long it takes to get pregnant?
● What is her experience of family and friends trying to conceive?
● What does her husband think about this?
● Did she and her husband use any form of contraception before they started trying for a baby?
● How long after stopping the combined pill did it take for her periods to return?
● Any previous pregnancies, miscarriages, terminations or pelvic surgery?
● Any previous sexually transmitted infections?
● Has she had any abdominal pains? Or vaginal discharge?
● Are her periods regular? Any bleeding between periods? Is her bleeding heavy?
● How often are they having sex? Is it vaginal sex?
● Is she still smoking? How much alcohol is she currently drinking?
● Does she take any regular medication, or over-the-counter or illicit drugs?
● Any family history of similar problems or early menopause?
● Does your husband have any children from previous relationships? Or has he ever made someone pregnant?
● What type of work does she do? And her husband? (Some occupational agents can have an effect on both women's and men's fertility – see NICE guideline reference).
● Does she know if she had a rubella vaccination when she was younger?

Domain 1 – Interpersonal skills

Offering reassurance

This patient has only been trying to get pregnant for 6 months and there is nothing in the history suggesting an underlying problem. The key here is to recognize her presentation as normal; explain this to the patient and try and reassure her, and then to go on to offer health promotion advice about trying to conceive:

- The patient has an unrealistic expectation of how long it normally takes to conceive. You could make clear that it is not unusual – even for normal healthy couples – to take a year, or longer, to conceive (see Knowledge-base).
- The patient and her husband have only been trying for 6 months and for the majority of that time it was difficult to have regular sex due to living with her parents-in-law.
- Also, it can take a few months after stopping the pill before the body returns to a normal hormonal cycle.
- However, she is now having regular periods, which suggests that she is ovulating – *'producing an egg that can join up with a sperm to make an embryo which grows into a baby.'* A diagram might help her understanding.
- As she and her husband have found out, it can be stressful trying to have sex at particular times each month. You should advise her that this is not necessary and they should just try to have regular sexual intercourse – about two to three times a week.
- You should explain that they (and it should ideally be both of them) only need to come back to the surgery if she is still not pregnant after a year in total of trying.

Domain 3 – Clinical management skills

Health promotion around fertility issues

You should use this opportunity to discuss lifestyle issues such as smoking, alcohol, diet, exercise and weight loss, which could all help increase the patient's chance of becoming pregnant, while also promoting general good health:

- Stopping smoking would be of huge benefit to her health, may increase her chance of conceiving and is important for a healthy pregnancy. Might this be something she and her husband would consider doing together so that the home environment becomes a smoke-free zone for their future child?
- Advise her to reduce her alcohol intake, down to a maximum of a half to one can of normal strength lager (1–2 units) a week, and avoid any episodes of intoxication. Does she think she would be able to do this?
- Women with a BMI > 29 are likely to take longer to conceive. You could discuss this with the patient and look at ways she might address this, including through her diet and taking more exercise.
- You have given the patient a lot of information today. If she has any further questions, or wants to talk more about this, then perhaps next time she could bring her husband too.

Knowledge-base – Infertility

Extract from: National Institute for Health and Clinical Excellence (NICE) (2004) CG 11. Fertility: assessment and treatment for people with fertility problems (clinical practice algorithm). London: NICE, February 2004. www.nice.org.uk. Reproduced with permission.

Infertility
Failure to conceive after regular unprotected sexual intercourse for 2 years in the absence of known reproductive pathology *This guideline does not include the management of people who are outside the definition, such as those with sexual dysfunction, couples who are using contraception and couples outside the reproductive age range*

Early investigation if:
• History of predisposing factors (such as amenorrhoea, oligomenorrhoea, pelvic inflammatory disease or undescended testes) • Woman's age ≥ 35 years • People with HIV, hepatitis B and hepatitis C • Prior treatment for cancer

Initial advice for people concerned about delays in conception:

• Cumulative probability of pregnancy in general population:
  ○ 84% in first year
  ○ 92% in second year
• Fertility declines with a woman's age
• Lifestyle advice:
  ○ Sexual intercourse every 2–3 days
  ○ ≤ 1–2 units alcohol once or twice a week for women; ≤ 3–4 units/day* for men
  ○ Smoking cessation programme for smokers
  ○ Body mass index of 19–29
  ○ Information about prescribed, over-the-counter and recreational drugs
  ○ Information about occupational hazards
• Offer preconceptional advice:
  ○ Folic acid
  ○ Rubella susceptibility and cervical screening

Principles of care:
• Couple-centred management • Access to evidence-based information (verbal and written) • Counselling from someone not directly involved in management of the couple's fertility problems • Contact with fertility support groups • Specialist teams

*The clinical practice algorithm actually states: '≥ 3–4 units/*week* for men', but this is an error (personal communication Iain Moir, NICE).

• Clinical investigation of fertility problems should not usually be necessary until couples have failed to conceive after 1 year of regular unprotected sexual intercourse.

Take home messages

- Patients' understanding of what constitutes 'normal' can be unrealistic.
- Patient education and providing reassurance are key roles for the GP.
- Use every opportunity for health promotion.

Ideas for further revision

It is easy to dismiss patients who present when there is no medical abnormality as the 'worried well'. However, as healthcare professionals we should see patient education and providing reassurance as key roles. These consultations also offer an opportunity to give healthy lifestyle advice. In your day-to-day surgeries, try and regularly offer such advice, such that this becomes almost second nature. Simple health promotion strategies, such as encouraging smoking cessation, offer patients an extremely cost-effective intervention.

Further reading

Infertility Network UK – advice and support for those dealing with fertility problems. www.infertilitynetworkuk.com.

NHS National Library for Health Clinical Knowledge Summaries – Infertility. http://cks.library.nhs.uk/.

NICE guideline – Fertility: assessment and treatment for people with fertility problems. CG11 February 2004. www.nice.org.uk.

RCGP curriculum statement 10.1 – Women's health. www.rcgp.org.uk.

Information given to candidates

Candidates note: This station is a **telephone consultation** with a patient. Please answer the telephone when it rings. The examiner will not enter your room, but will be able to hear both you and the patient.

Miranda Rogerson is a 42-year-old female patient with Crohn's disease.

She has been under the care of the gastroenterologists for 4 years.

The last clinic letter from 1 month ago states:

Dear GP,

Mrs Rogerson is currently stable on azathioprine 125 mg OD. However, she has had three admissions in the last year with flare ups of her colonic inflammatory Crohn's disease and her last colonoscopy revealed a well defined region in the proximal ascending colon. We have discussed with Mrs Rogerson that surgery will probably be the next option if things flare up again, although we would of course reassess at that time.'

The patient's GP surgery – where you are based – is in London.

The first thing the patient says when you pick up the phone is, "Hello doctor, it's Miranda Rogerson here. I'm away on business at the moment in Aberdeen and the Crohn's seems to be flaring up."

- What do you think this station is testing?
- Make notes or discuss your thoughts with a colleague before you read on.

Plan your approach to this station:

Information given to simulated patient

Basic details – You are Miranda Rogerson, a Caucasian 42-year-old management consultant currently on a week-long visit to one of your clients in Aberdeen. You are ringing your GP surgery back in London for advice. You suffer from Crohn's disease (an inflammatory condition affecting your bowels) which seems to have flared up in the last 3 days.

Appearance and behaviour – You come across on the telephone as articulate and intelligent. Initially you underplay the severity of your symptoms, to try and persuade the doctor – and yourself – that you can wait until you return home before you see someone.

History
Freely divulged to doctor – You have Crohn's disease and see the specialist team at your local hospital in London every 4 months. Things have been fairly settled since you were last discharged from hospital 4 months ago, after a week's stay. You take regular medication to 'keep on top of the Crohn's'. You have not been feeling too good for 3 days, with diarrhoea and tummy pains.

Divulged to doctor if specifically asked – Yesterday you opened your bowels six times, and today you have been eight times already. The rectal bleeding you get when your Crohn's flares up is back and now pretty heavy (you have used four pads so far today). Your appetite has been poor for a couple of weeks and you have lost about 4 kg over that time. You have felt generally 'washed out' over the last week. You were feeling hot last night, and have taken plenty of paracetamol, but still feel feverish today. The abdominal pains are on the right hand side, lower down and it is particularly tender in that area. One of your colleagues said you were looking rather pale yesterday. You have not had any joint or eye problems.

Ideas, concerns and expectations – The work in Aberdeen is a key contract and you see it as a real opportunity to show your boss that you are ready for promotion. You feel that if you have to leave before the end of the week then it will not look good to your seniors. You know that your Crohn's is worse but you are hoping that you can hold out until the end of the trip. However, with the bleeding being so heavy you thought you should speak with the GP for advice. You are hoping that the doctor will arrange an appointment for you to see your specialist as soon as you get back, and sanction your plan to hold on until then. Another option you have considered is flying home today and going to your local hospital. However, if the doctor is understanding about your work predicament but explains the seriousness of your symptoms and the need for immediate assessment, then you will agree to go to the nearest A&E today.

First words spoken to doctor – "Hello doctor, it's Miranda Rogerson. I'm away on business at the moment in Aberdeen and the Crohn's seems to be flaring up".

Past medical history – You were diagnosed with Crohn's disease 4 years ago. You are otherwise fit and well. Things had been fairly stable for the first 3 years until you were admitted three times in the last year for your Crohn's disease, with each admission lasting about a week and requiring steroid treatment. Since the last discharge, 4 months ago, you have been doing well. However, your specialist has said that if you have any further flare ups then surgery may be the next option.

Drug history – You take five 25 mg tablets of azathioprine, once a day. You have no allergies.

Social history – You have a high-powered job working for a management consultancy firm in London. You stopped smoking when you were diagnosed with Crohn's disease 4 years ago. You live with your husband. You do not have any children.

Family history – Your maternal aunt has Crohn's disease. There are no other significant medical problems in your immediate family.

- Having read the information given to the simulated patient, what do you now think this station is testing?
- Make notes or discuss your thoughts with a colleague before you turn the page.

Review your approach to this station:

Tested at this station:

1. Interpersonal skills using the telephone
2. History taking skills
3. Negotiating a shared management plan

Domain I – Interpersonal skills

Interpersonal skills using the telephone

You need to be able to demonstrate that you are competent at conducting a consultation by telephone:

- A telephone consultation can seem relatively anonymous, so it is important to identify yourself and the patient, by name, to help build rapport.
- If there is any doubt as to the identity of the person you are speaking to, then arrange to call the patient back on a number documented in their medical notes.
- One way to conceptualize how best to conduct a telephone consultation is to think about best practice in communication skills for face-to-face encounters, then accentuate these. This strategy aims to help compensate for the visual information 'lost' in such an exchange – e.g.:
  - Use plenty of active listening noises or words – 'uh-huh', 'yes', 'right', etc.
  - Summarize regularly.
  - Repeatedly clarify the patient's ideas, concerns and expectations, so that you ensure that you address the patient's agenda.
  - Regularly 'chunk and check' – give small amounts of information then ask the patient to clarify what has been said – as they too will not have access to visual reminders or prompts.
  - Ensure that the patient is clearly in agreement with any management plan reached.

Domain 2 – Data gathering, examination and clinical assessment skills

History taking skills

Without visual cues from a face-to-face consultation and the inability to conduct a physical examination, it is all the more important that you take a detailed history:

- As with a face-to-face consultation, start with open questions. What has been happening with her health recently? What has prompted her to call today? What was she hoping you could do for her?
- With telephone consultations it is useful to find out the social context in which the patient is calling. In this case she is away from home on business and feels under pressure to delay attending hospital.
- The patient is reluctant to disclose the true severity of her symptoms. Asking specific closed questions will allow you to perform an appropriate assessment:

- How many times is she opening her bowels at the moment? How does this compare to normal?
- Are the stools well formed or loose?
- Any blood in the stools? How much? Has she had to use any pads?
- Has she vomited?
- What is her appetite like? Any weight loss recently?
- Does she feel feverish?
- Any abdominal pain? (see Examination 2: Station 6 – Knowledge-base.) How does it compare to when she was admitted to hospital?
- Any abdominal tenderness or bloating?
- It would also be important to obtain information on her current medication and any analgesia she is taking.

Domain 3 – Clinical management skills

Negotiating a shared management plan

The patient herself knows that she should really be properly assessed in hospital, but is trying to put this off for a few more days:

- Acknowledge the patient's perspective on events – she has a strong desire not to interrupt her current work commitments.
- However, make sure that you clearly state the seriousness of her condition – her Crohn's disease appears to be flaring up and the fever, rectal bleeding and tender abdomen are all worrying signs. Does she recognize this?
- The current picture suggests a serious complication of Crohn's disease, such as toxic dilatation (dangerous swelling up of her bowel), perforation of the bowel or abscess formation. If she decides not to go to hospital today, then she must realize that these are all potentially life-threatening conditions.
- If she suggests coming home today, to go to her local hospital, then you should point out that even this delay could prove disastrous if she suddenly deteriorates en route.
- Your advice to her must be that she needs to be assessed without delay and started on appropriate treatment.
- You could suggest that if she went into hospital in Aberdeen they could easily call you and her London specialist for further information.
- Knowing all this, what does she want to do?

Knowledge-base – Suggested approach to a telephone consultation

- Answer the telephone promptly
- State your name
- Obtain the caller's name and telephone number (in case the patient has to be called back by another member of the team or the call is disconnected)
- Speak directly with the person who has a problem
- Record the date and time of the call
- Record the person's name, sex and age (obtain medical records if available)
- Take a detailed and structured history

- Provide advice on treatment or disposition
- Advise about follow-up and when to contact the doctor (e.g. worsening symptoms despite treatment, symptoms failing to improve within a week, onset of new symptoms)
- Summarize the main points covered
- Request the caller to repeat the advice given (several times throughout the consultation)
- Ask if the person has any outstanding questions or concerns
- Let the caller disconnect first

From: Car & Sheikh (2003). Reproduced with permission from BMJ Publishing Group.

Take home messages

- Telephone consultations deprive you of a wealth of visual information available from face-to-face meetings and therefore require you to take a particularly thorough history.
- If you feel unhappy agreeing to a course of action without seeing the patient, then arrange for a face-to-face contact, either with yourself or another healthcare professional.
- When agreeing a management plan with a patient on the telephone, ensure that safety-netting and follow-up are clearly understood.

Ideas for further revision

The CSA can assess various ways of communicating with patients, such as through a third party, by telephone or with an interpreter. Think about, and practise, how you might adapt your consultation style to meet these communication challenges.

Further reading

British Society of Gastroenterology. Guidelines for the management of inflammatory bowel disease in adults, 2004. www.bsg.org.uk.

Car J, Sheikh A. Telephone consultations. *BMJ* 2003;**326**:966–969. www.bmj.com.

Males T. *Telephone Consultations in Primary Care – A Practical Guide.* London: Royal College of General Practitioners, 2007.

NHS National Library for Health Clinical Knowledge Summaries – Crohn's disease. www.cks.library.nhs.uk/clinical_knowledge.

RCGP curriculum statement 15.2 – Clinical Management: Digestive problems. www.rcgp.org.uk.

Examination 1: Station 13

Information given to candidates

Stephanie Browne is a 46-year-old woman who rarely comes to the surgery.

You note that she saw a colleague 8 years ago with acute low back pain, which settled with conservative treatment within a month.

Her only other past medical history includes mild indigestion, for which she takes over-the-counter antacid medication.

Before surgery today one of the receptionists commented that Ms Browne 'can be very talkative' and joked that she didn't think Ms Browne would be in the consultation room with you for less than half an hour.

The patient enters the room walking slowly with her left hand on her lumbar spine.

- What do you think this station is testing?
- Make notes or discuss your thoughts with a colleague before you read on.

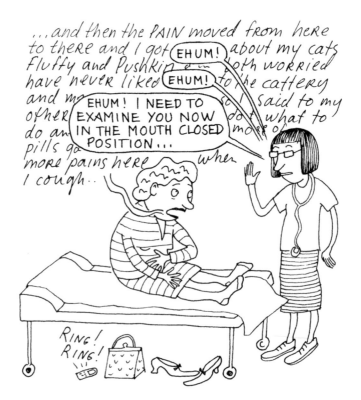

Plan your approach to this station:

Information given to simulated patient

Basic details – You are Stephanie Browne, a Caucasian 46-year-old woman who works for a small local business selling double-glazing.

Appearance and behaviour – You are naturally a talkative person and are inclined to talk at length during the consultation. You fill the silences even during any examination the doctor may perform. During the consultation you often find yourself digressing in your answers. On several occasions you will need the doctor politely to interrupt you if you are to be focused back to answering the questions they have asked.

History
Freely divulged to doctor – Two days ago you were lifting a heavy box at home in an awkward twisted position. As you started to lift you felt a sharp pain in your lower back on the left hand side. You dropped the box. You were able to walk to the couch nearby and then lay down very carefully due to the pain. Your lower back seemed to 'seize up' and it was very painful if you tried to move.

Divulged to doctor if specifically asked – The pain is much more bearable if you lie still. You have been resting on the couch and then in bed since the injury happened. You have not had any problems passing urine or opening your bowels. You have not had any pains in your legs or any numbness or weakness. You have not felt any pins and needles in your buttocks or lower back and your sensation has been normal. Other than the pain you feel well in yourself. You have not been feverish. You have taken the occasional paracetamol for the pain but did not want to take too many tablets before seeing the doctor. Your mood is usually fine and even with this setback you are 'not too down in the dumps' about it as it got better last time and so you think the same thing should happen again.

Ideas, concerns and expectations – You were told that bed rest was the best thing for back pain when you hurt your back in a similar way 8 years ago, so you have been following this advice since the recent injury. Because the pain is not too bad if you are lying down, you believe that bringing the pain on by getting up and about must be harmful. However, if the doctor explains in a supportive and understanding manner, how staying mobile is the best thing for your back, then you will be responsive to this advice. You have been worrying about your cats as on a couple of occasions you felt in too much pain when trying to get up to feed them, and so they went hungry. You want to know how long the problem will last and whether you should put them in the cattery.

First words spoken to doctor – "I've hurt my back and the pain has been terrible doctor."

Past medical history – You had a similar episode of sudden onset lower back pain 8 years ago when you were moving house and helping your brother lift a table. However, your back has not really bothered you since that episode. You broke your left arm when you were 10 years old when you fell off a wall, but have not fractured any bones since then. You suffer from indigestion after large evening meals.

Drug history – You take Rennies for indigestion about once a week. You are not allergic to any medication.

Social history – You work for a small local double-glazing firm in their sales office telephoning potential customers. This involves sitting at a computer for most of the day. You live on your own with three cats that are much more than just pets to you. You enjoy gardening and used to walk the 1½ miles to work, although for the last 6 months you have been taking the bus. You have some good friends nearby and one younger brother who has his own young family, who you get on well with. You stopped smoking 15 years ago and drink the odd glass of wine with meals.

Family history – There are no serious medical problems in your immediate family.

- Having read the information given to the simulated patient, what do you now think this station is testing?
- Make notes or discuss your thoughts with a colleague before you turn the page.

Review your approach to this station:

Tested at this station:

1. Dealing with a talkative patient
2. Data gathering
3. Excluding serious pathology
4. Physical examination
5. Management of common medical conditions presenting in primary care

Domain I – Interpersonal skills

Dealing with a talkative patient

In the CSA you only have 10 min for each consultation and there is often a fair amount to cover with each patient. Unless you manage talkative patients appropriately, then you will run out of time and lose marks:

- In real life, many patients have a 'script' of what they want to say to the doctor, which they have rehearsed in the waiting room. Letting patients speak uninterrupted initially allows you to gather key details from the history and lets patients disclose their agenda.
- Thereafter, it is important for the doctor to take control and direct the consultation to ensure that all the main issues are covered adequately.
- Talkative patients can present a challenge to this consultation method and need to be politely, but firmly, steered back to the key points.
- One tactic is to acknowledge any digressions, and then focus the patient back to the question asked – e.g. *"You are obviously worried about your cats and I can see that they are important to you, but if I can just be clear about your back pain…is the pain going down into your legs?"*
- Another tactic is regularly to summarize problems and concerns to allow you to impose some focus to the consultation.
- If you need to interrupt patients, then use non-verbal as well as verbal signs, such as raising your hand, to indicate that you need to speak.
- Patients often want to continue the discussion when you are examining them. This may allow you to multitask and gain valuable additional information, although be wary of such interactions stalling the examination process.

Domain 2 – Data gathering, examination and clinical assessment skills

Data gathering

Although the majority of acute back pain episodes resolve within a few weeks, it is important to take an adequate history to exclude serious conditions:

- History taking:
  - How did the patient sustain the injury?
  - How has she been managing since the injury?
  - Has there been any recent history of trauma?
  - Has she had back problems before?
  - Can she describe the pain – its site, nature, severity and if it radiates?

- Does she have any pain, numbness or altered sensation in her legs?
- What makes the pain better and what makes it worse?
- Has she been taking anything for the pain?
- Does the patient suffer from osteoporosis ('thin bones')?
- Any previous fractured bones?
- Any past medical history of cancer?
- Yellow flags – these represent psychosocial features associated with progression to chronic problems and disability:
  - Is the patient reluctant to do anything that brings on the pain as she thinks that this is harmful?
  - Does she fear the pain and is this fear making her increasingly inactive?
  - Is she more inclined to think that passive – as opposed to active – treatment will help?
  - How is her mood? Is she anxious, stressed or socially withdrawn?
  - Any financial or social problems?
  - Is there a history of problems at work?
  - Is her family overprotective?
  - An exaggerated response to examination can also be a yellow flag.

Excluding serious pathology

Red flags or indications for immediate admission must be excluded before you allow patients with acute back pain to leave the consulting room:

- Emergency action required – symptoms or signs suggestive of cauda equina syndrome or rapidly progressing neurological deficit would require immediate referral, including:
  - Saddle anaesthesia
  - Recent onset of bladder or bowel problems – particularly urinary retention or bowel incontinence
  - Gait problems.
- Red flags – may indicate serious spinal pathology:
  - Age of first presentation < 20 or > 50 years old
  - Past medical history of cancer
  - Systemically unwell – e.g. fever, weight loss
  - Thoracic back pain
  - Pain worse if lying down
  - Severe pain at night
  - Intravenous drug use
  - Protracted steroid use.
- If any red flags present then consider investigations including FBC, ESR, urinalysis, X-ray, bone scan or referral.

Physical examination skills

Information from a brief, but focused, clinical examination in combination with the history helps categorize the cause of back pain:

- Any asymmetry on inspection? – e.g. scoliosis.
- Where exactly is the pain – is it definitely in the lower back rather than, say, the hips?

- Any spinal tenderness on palpation? – e.g. in vertebral collapse.
- Any reduction in spinal range of movement? – flexion, extension, lateral flexion and rotation.
- Assess power in legs – any weakness in knee extension, foot dorsiflexion or ankle eversion?
- Assess lower limb reflexes.
- Assess sensation – if there is a deficit, what is the distribution?
- Straight leg raises – any reduction? Unilateral or bilateral? Sciatic stretch test positive (dorsiflexion of foot increases any leg pain)?
- Do not forget to assess the patient as she walks into the consultation room and manoeuvres herself onto the examination couch
- In the rare event of suspecting cauda equina syndrome, a PR examination would be indicated, but this is not necessary here, and you would never be expected to perform such an examination on a simulated patient in the CSA (although you might have to do so on a model).

Domain 3 – Clinical management skills

Management of common medical conditions presenting in primary care

Appropriate advice and analgesia will aid this patient's recovery from her episode of acute simple (mechanical) lower back pain:

- General advice to help improve long term back health, including:
  - Posture – could she improve the set-up of her chair, desk and computer at work?
  - Increased activity levels – maybe she could restart walking the 1½ miles to work again rather than taking the bus?
  - Proper lifting techniques – she has injured her back twice through lifting heavy objects – does she know to bend her knees not her back?
- There are no worrying signs or symptoms and your working diagnosis should be simple (mechanical) lower back pain. Explain that the cause is probably a strain of a muscle and reassure the patient that a full recovery is likely.
- Explain that our understanding of what is best for this sort of back pain has changed and encourage her to stay mobile rather than taking to bed.
- She should aim to get back to work at the earliest opportunity to aid recovery.
- Prognosis and reassurance – you can advise her that in 9 of 10 patients with this problem the pain has gone or significantly improved within 6 weeks.
- Regular analgesia, rather than PRN, such as paracetamol 1 g QDS and a NSAID, such as ibuprofen 400 mg TDS, would usually be recommended. However, this patient suffers from indigestion so you should either co-prescribe a PPI with the NSAID or replace the NSAID with a weak opiate.
- Given her description of her lower back 'seizing up', you may want to consider a short course of PRN muscle relaxant – e.g. diazepam 2 mg TDS – to help ease any acute muscle spasm.
- Ask her to return in 6 weeks if things are not improving, or sooner if she has any new symptoms or concerns.

Knowledge-base – Back pain

References – See Further reading.

	Features	*Management*
Simple (mechanical) back pain	• Pain worse on movement • Pain worse after sitting or standing for long periods • No red flags • May be precipitating injury – e.g. lifting heavy object • Reduced range of movement of spine due to pain • Dull ache may radiate to buttocks or thighs	• Adequate analgesia: regular paracetamol and NSAIDs, unless contraindicated • Encourage the patient to stay mobile and return to work – with modifications if indicated • Inform patients about manipulation options – physiotherapy, osteopathy and chiropractic • Consider muscle relaxants – e.g. diazepam • X-rays not usually indicated
Nerve root pain	• As for simple (mechanical) back pain, but leg pain is often sharp and well localized • Leg pain – can be worse than any associated back pain • Straight leg raises reduced and stretch test positive • May be abnormal reflexes – e.g. absent ankle jerk, and/ or altered sensation – e.g. numbness or parasthesia	• As for simple (mechanical) back pain, plus: • Reassure that conservative treatment should be adequate • Advise may take 6–8 weeks for full recovery
Inflammatory causes of back pain	• Ankylosing spondylitis – back pain worse in morning or after inactivity • Rheumatoid arthritis (RA) – often multiple joints affected • Osteoarthritis (OA) – usually older age onset than RA	• X-rays of spine and pelvis and HLA-B27 antigen test for suspected ankylosing spondylitis • Rheumatoid factor, FBC and ESR if RA suspected, plus referral to rheumatology and analgesia • Adequate analgesia and lifestyle advice for OA
More serious causes of back pain	• Cauda equina syndrome • Aortic aneurysm • Myeloma • Vertebral collapse – secondary to osteoporosis or malignancy	• Immediate referral required for suspected cauda equina syndrome or aortic aneurysm • X-rays for suspected myeloma plus urine for Bence Jones protein and blood tests – including ESR and serum protein electrophoresis • X-rays for suspected vertebral collapse plus FBC, calcium and LFTs, and adequate analgesia

- If simple (mechanical) back pain is not improving after 6 weeks then reconsider diagnosis – investigations may include FBC, alkaline phosphatase, ESR and calcium.
- Chronic back pain is defined as pain lasting longer than 12 weeks.

Take home messages

- With talkative patients, take control of the consultation and politely, but firmly, steer them back to the key issues.
- In back pain, be alert to red flags or any neurological findings that require immediate referral.
- In simple (mechanical) back pain encourage early return to normal activities to aid recovery.

Ideas for further revision

Time constraints in the CSA can make some stations particularly challenging. In the weeks before you take this assessment try getting your consultations down to 10 min, to allow you to feel familiar and confident with consulting within this time frame.

Further reading

European guidelines for the management of acute non-specific low back pain in primary care. European Commission. Research Directorate General 2004. www.backpaineurope.org/web/files/WG1_Guidelines.pdf.

New Zealand Acute Low Back Pain Guide – Incorporating the guide to assessing the psychosocial yellow flags in acute low back pain, 2002. www. nzgg.org.nz/guidelines/0072/acc1038_col.pdf.

NHS National Library for Health Clinical Knowledge Summaries: Back pain – lower. www.cks.library.nhs.uk/clinical_knowledge.

RCGP curriculum statement 15.9 – Clinical management: Rheumatology & conditions of the musculoskeletal system (including trauma). www.rcgp.org.uk.

Samanta J, Kendall J, Samanta A. 10-minute consultation: Chronic low back pain. *BMJ* 2003;**326**:535.

Examination 2

Stations 1–13

Examination 2: Station 1

Information given to candidates

> George Agnew is a 72-year-old patient who lives with his long-term partner, Hilary. George has asked for an appointment to talk about his concerns regarding Hilary's health. George is attending on his own today.

As George enters the consulting room he says, "I'm concerned that Hilary's memory seems to be going. I think it might be the beginnings of Alzheimer's. After 30 years together I'm worried our relationship is breaking down."

- What do you think this station is testing?
- Make notes or discuss your thoughts with a colleague before you read on.

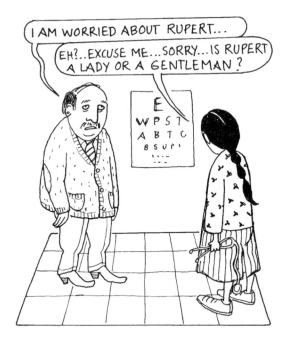

Plan your approach to this station:

Information given to simulated carer

Basic details – You are George Agnew, a Caucasian 72-year-old retired school-teacher. You have come to the surgery to discuss your concerns regarding the health of your long-term male partner, Hilary Mendle, who is 68 years old.

Appearance and behaviour – You are well presented, wearing a jacket and tie. You are a little anxious as you believe that seeing the doctor today will probably set in train a series of events that will take matters partly out of your hands. In some sense, you are relieved at this, having been carrying around for some time now your own 'secret' – namely your fear that Hilary is showing signs of 'Alzheimer's'.

History

Freely divulged to doctor – Hilary's memory started to get worse about a year ago. There has been a gradual decline over that time. Now he needs to write lists to remind himself about even the smallest thing. More recently, he has been forgetting the way home from the local shops and on two occasions you had to go out to find him wandering nearby. He used to be a keen letter writer but now finds it difficult even to write a short postcard. He gets confused in new surroundings. Your friends have started to comment.

Divulged to doctor if specifically asked – He has never been an aggressive man, but last week Hilary became agitated and upset at home after you had rearranged the furniture in the front room, and he smashed one of your treasured school photos. You were shocked when he did not recognize some old friends of you both when you bumped into them in the supermarket. Hilary has been well in himself otherwise – no chesty coughs or complaints of any pains. He has never smoked. Hilary does seem to recognize the problems he is having with his memory, but he dismisses it as 'just old age'. He got quite angry when you suggested coming to see the doctor today as he denied that anything was wrong. Hilary does not drive. You are now having to do most of the household chores yourself.

Ideas, concerns and expectations – You have been putting off coming to see the doctor for several months as you did not want to accept what was happening. You have been together for over 30 years and feel that you would not know how to cope if, as you fear, a diagnosis of Alzheimer's disease is made. Both of you have always been very private people and the idea of having to explain your domestic situation 'to strangers' from numerous agencies who might be involved in Hilary's care is something you worry about greatly. The recent aggressive episodes did really worry you, and prompted you to attend today. You want to know if there is anything that can be done to help with these in particular. You suspect that the doctor will talk about Hilary having to go into a residential home but you want him to stay at home as long as he can. You want to know how long it will be before he stops recognizing you. You have heard about medication that can help and want to ask the doctor about this.

First words spoken to doctor – "I'm concerned that Hilary's memory seems to be going. I think it might be the beginnings of Alzheimer's. After 30 years together I'm worried our relationship is breaking down."

Past medical history – You are in good physical health and only take a daily aspirin. Hilary has been a fit and active man all his life and apart from a hip replacement 2 years ago has been 'in rude health'.

Drug history – Hilary takes the odd painkiller for arthritis but does not have any regular medication.

Social history – You both worked as teachers in private schools until you both retired 7 years ago. You met Hilary 30 years ago at a teaching conference and have been living together since then. Your respective families never inquired in too much detail about your relationship and over time you have both lost touch with them. You were both active in your retirement, travelling abroad and playing bridge for the local club.

Family history – As far as you are aware, there are no major health problems in Hilary's family.

- Having read the information given to the simulated carer, what do you now think this station is testing?
- Make notes or discuss your thoughts with a colleague before you turn the page.

Review your approach to this station:

Tested at this station:

1. Understanding of equality and diversity issues
2. Taking a history from a third party
3. Supporting a patient's carer

Domain 1 – Interpersonal skills

Understanding of equality and diversity issues

The new GP curriculum states that promoting equality and valuing diversity are at the heart of the curriculum, and that diversity is about recognizing and valuing difference in its broadest sense. The carer in this scenario happens to be in a same-sex relationship. You need to avoid being judgemental or making assumptions that could lead to a breakdown of trust within the consultation:

- When patients, relatives or carers use gender neutral terms such as 'partner', be alert to the fact that they could be referring to a same-sex partner.
- Do not make assumptions regarding the sexual orientation of a patient, carer or relative. If you get it wrong (e.g. by asking about a male patient's 'wife' or 'girlfriend' when his partner is male), some patients may decide not to correct you but will feel that you are not a doctor who could be responsive to their needs, and may simply book again to see someone else.
- If you do get it wrong and are corrected by the patient, carer or relative, although you may be embarrassed at your error, it is best just to apologize for your mistake and move on.
- You may have strong personal beliefs around sexuality issues, but in your role as a medical practitioner you need to be non-judgemental and remain professional.
- In the new edition of *Good Medical Practice*, the General Medical Council makes clear that the duties of a doctor include never discriminating unfairly against patients or colleagues by allowing personal views on issues such as sexual orientation to adversely affect professional relationships with them (paragraph 7 – see Further reading).
- In this scenario, being accepting and understanding of the worries George has regarding potentially having to disclose his and Hilary's domestic situation to numerous outside agencies – 'to strangers' – is a key skill that will allow you to demonstrate your awareness of equality and diversity issues to the examiner.

Domain 2 – Data gathering, examination and clinical assessment skills

Taking a history from a third party

In many circumstances taking a history from someone who is not the patient can be problematical, but when the presenting complaint is memory difficulties and aggressive behaviour it is essential to have a clear history from a third party:

- When did George first notice problems with Hilary's memory? Can he give examples? How have things progressed? Has anyone else commented on this?
- Have the changes been gradual or stepwise?
- Has Hilary's personality changed in any way?
- Hilary was aggressive last week, and this was out of character for him. When and where did this episode occur – e.g. was it at dusk? Were there any obvious triggers? Has Hilary been unwell over the last week – e.g. with a chesty cough or going to the toilet more frequently to urinate?
- Has Hilary been complaining of any other problems – any pains, weight loss or low mood?
- Have there been any episodes where Hilary has put himself – or others – in danger, e.g. leaving the gas on?
- Does Hilary suffer from any other medical conditions, such as diabetes or high blood pressure?
- Does he take any medication? Has he started any new medicines over the last year?
- Has Hilary ever had a heart attack or stroke?
- Does he smoke?
- Does Hilary drive?
- What does Hilary think about what has been happening? Does he recognize that there is a problem?
- Is there a reason why George has come on his own? Does Hilary know that George is here today?

Domain 3 – Clinical management skills

Supporting a patient's carer

George has come to you today to seek help and support regarding his concerns about Hilary. You need to provide genuine support to George as a carer by acknowledging his worries, exploring his own feelings about the situation and providing information on what will happen next:

- Thank George for coming to see you today and explain how the information he is able to give about Hilary is extremely useful.
- Empathize that it must have been very difficult to carry on for so long without discussing his concerns with anyone else.
- George is fairly convinced that Hilary has Alzheimer's disease. Why does he think this? Has he had previous experience of people with dementia?
- What are George's thoughts about what will happen next? Does he have any specific worries or concerns?
- Hilary does seem to have some idea that his memory is worsening, but he dismisses it as 'just old age'. What does George think about this? Might Hilary be using denial as a coping strategy?
- Explain that there could be a number of different causes of Hilary's symptoms (e.g. depression, the effect of medication or other medical problems such as hormone or vitamin deficiencies) and that a diagnosis would only be made after a proper assessment.
- Hilary refused to come to the surgery today, but would he accept a home visit? If Hilary is adamant that he will not see a doctor, then you would

need to explain to George how it is difficult for you to go against Hilary's expressed wishes.

- Explain that if Hilary allows you to visit, you will do some simple memory tests and may need to take blood to exclude various physical causes. If appropriate, you may end up referring him to the memory clinic for further specialist assessment.
- Advise George that Hilary will be involved in all stages of the investigation process. Explain how you would ask Hilary how much he wanted to know about his problem, and would never force information on him against his wishes.
- Advise George that, if a diagnosis of dementia is subsequently made, there are support services available for carers including:
  ○ Provision of home care packages to support patients in their own home.
  ○ Psychological therapies available for carers.
  ○ Carer support groups and carer training programmes.
  ○ Respite care.
  ○ Input from district nurses to give advice about nursing care.
  ○ Support from community psychiatric nurses.
  ○ Age Concern – the UK's largest organization working with and for older people – has local support groups and a useful website aimed at carers too (see Further reading).
- George is particularly worried about the recent aggressiveness. Explain that there may be a number of reasons for this, e.g. an infection or the recent change to a familiar environment that has upset him. Say that you can assess this when you visit, but that there are therapies available to deal with such challenging behaviour (see Knowledge-base). Advise George not to make any changes about the house or to their routines at the moment.

Knowledge-base – Dementia

References – see Further reading.

Definition	A global impairment of cognitive function without clouding of consciousness
Living with dementia	• 1 in 20 aged > 65 years • 1 in 5 aged > 80 years
Types	• Alzheimer's disease – most common form (approximately 60%) • Vascular dementia – progression may be stepwise (approximately 20%) • Lewy body dementia – can have hallucinations and Parkinsonism, e.g. tremors and bradykinesia • Frontotemporal lobe dementia – rare, includes Pick's disease, often affects those < 65 years old. Memory may be intact but personality can change
Investigations	• Appropriate history and examination to exclude other causes – e.g. depression, medication, other medical conditions • MMSE – Mini-Mental State Examination 30 point formal cognitive test or abbreviated tools, such as the AMTS – Abbreviated Mental Test Score • Blood tests – FBC, U&Es, TFTs, glucose, LFTs, Ca, B_{12} and folate • MSU, CXR and consider ECG (some memory clinics request this routinely) • NICE recommends not routinely testing for syphilis or HIV, unless indicated
Referral	To specialist memory clinics for further assessment of cognitive, behavioural and global functioning by elderly care psychiatry teams. Imaging may subsequently be arranged (e.g. MRI)
Interventions	• Acetylcholinesterase inhibitors (e.g. donepezil, galantamine, rivastigmine) may be considered as adjunct treatment for Alzheimer's disease • Review and treat vascular risk factors • Care plans to maximize independent activity and help support carers • Reality orientation – regularly orientating people in time, place and key facts • For challenging behaviour – address environmental and psychosocial factors. NICE lists non-pharmacological interventions including: aromatherapy, massage, music and dance therapy, and multisensory stimulation

Mental Capacity Act 2005 for England and Wales	• Came into force in April 2007
	• A statutory framework to empower and protect those who may lack capacity to make decisions for themselves
	• Adults presumed to have capacity unless proven otherwise
	• Individuals must be given all practicable support before it is concluded that they are not able to make their own decisions
	• Individuals are able to make what might be seen as an unwise decision
	• Anything done for or on behalf of individuals without capacity:
	  ○ Must be in their best interests
	  ○ Should restrict their rights and basic freedoms as little as possible.
	• Lasting Powers of Attorney – individuals can appoint someone to make health and welfare decisions on their behalf, if they lose capacity at some future time.

Take home messages

- Avoid making assumptions about people's sexual orientation.
- Only in exceptional circumstances should you go against the express wishes of patients.
- Thorough assessment is required of anyone presenting with cognitive impairment.
- Supporting carers is a key role of the primary healthcare team.

Ideas for further revision

Your local mental health unit should have a memory clinic run by the elderly care psychiatry team. Arrange to spend some time with them sitting in on clinics and speaking to members of the multidisciplinary team. Find out what they expect of primary care before patients are referred with suspected dementia to specialist services.

Further reading

Alzheimer's Disease Society. www.alzheimers.org.uk.

Breen DA, Breen DP, Moore JW, Breen PA, O'Neill D. Driving and dementia. *BMJ* 2007;**334**:1365–1369. www.bmj.com.

Department of Health information leaflet – An introduction to working with lesbian, gay and bisexual people: information for health and social care staff. April 2007. www.dh.gov.uk/en/Publicationsandstatistics/Publications/PublicationsPolicyAndGuidance/DH_074255.

General Medical Council. *Good Medical Practice.* London: GMC, 2006. www.gmc-uk.org/guidance/good_medical_practice/index.asp.

Kai J (ed). *Valuing Diversity – A Resource for Effective Health Care of Ethnically Diverse Communities – A Training Manual.* London: Royal College of General Practitioners, 2004.

Mental Capacity Act 2005. www.dca.gov.uk/menincap/legis.htm.

NICE guidelines 42. Dementia: Supporting people with dementia and their carers in health and social care. November 2006. http://guidance.nice.org.uk/cg41.

RCGP curriculum statement 9 – Care of older adults. www.rcgp.org.uk.

Scottish Intercollegiate Guidelines Network (SIGN) guidelines 86. Management of patients with dementia, February 2006. www.sign.ac.uk/pdf/sign86.pdf.

Examination 2: Station 2

Information given to candidates

Sarah Chatwich is a 42-year-old patient who rarely comes to the surgery. Previous entries in her records are for smears and minor illnesses.

A pop-up box on her computer records reminds you that she has impaired hearing and lip reads.

As the patient enters the room she says, "I've been feeling so tired and run down recently doctor – I'm worried there's something seriously wrong."

- What do you think this station is testing?
- Make notes or discuss your thoughts with a colleague before you read on.

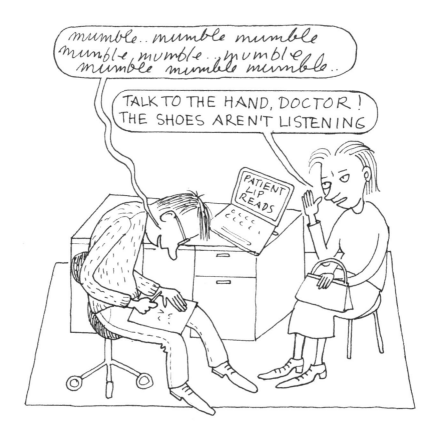

Plan your approach to this station:

Information given to simulated patient

Basic details – You are Sarah Chatwich, a Caucasian 42-year-old single woman who works full-time as a manager in an IT (computer) firm.

Appearance and behaviour – You are well presented. You wear hearing aids in both ears. You have minimal hearing and understand people primarily by lip reading. Consequently, you need to have a clear view of the doctor's face. You will miss what is being said unless the doctor speaks slowly and clearly, and faces you when speaking. You get annoyed if people patronize you because of your hearing impairment and you will challenge the doctor if you feel that their behaviour is inappropriate in this regard.

History

Freely divulged to doctor – You have been feeling run down for several months now. You are tired all the time and lack energy. When you were on holiday in the USA recently, your American friend said that you might have a hormone problem and that you should see your doctor when you got home. You are putting on weight – about a stone over the last year, despite trying to eat a healthy diet. When in America, even though the weather was fairly warm, you found yourself wearing more layers than the rest of your group, and looking back you have been feeling the cold more for a while.

Divulged to doctor if specifically asked – Your periods are regular but have been getting heavier over recent months. You get constipated – something you never used to suffer from – with hard stools and you are now only opening your bowels twice a week (last year you used to go almost every day). You feel as though you have been slowed down over the last 3 or 4 months, and you sometimes find it difficult to concentrate on things, but you put this down to being so tired. You have not felt depressed. You have no problems sleeping or with your appetite. You are not going to the toilet to urinate more frequently and you are not excessively thirsty. You have never suffered from chest pain or had any heart problems. You have never suffered from high blood pressure or headaches.

Ideas, concerns and expectations – To begin with you just put down your symptoms to being run down due to work pressures, but as things have got worse you are now worried that there may be something seriously wrong, although you are not sure what this could be. Your American friend's comments have further reinforced your concerns. You want the doctor to try and get to the bottom of things.

First words spoken to doctor – "I've been feeling so tired and run down recently doctor – I'm worried there's something seriously wrong."

Past medical history – You lost most of your hearing when you were 4 years old and were told this was the result of a severe infection. You have worn hearing aids since then and this has allowed you to maintain your speech, such that you speak almost as clearly as someone without any hearing impairment. You rarely come to see the doctor, other than for smears and minor problems. You have never been depressed.

Drug history – You do not take any regular medication. You do not have any drug allergies.

Social history – You were discouraged from learning sign language when you were a child as your parents were advised that you would be more likely to integrate into a mainstream school if you were forced to lip read. You have never really had any friends within the deaf community. You have never smoked and drink one or two glasses of wine each day over the weekend. You live with Rex, your Labrador.

Family history – Your mother had diabetes mellitus, requiring tablets from when she was diagnosed in her 40s. She died aged 62 from a stroke. Your father and brother are fit and well. As far as you know, no-one in your family has had heart or cholesterol problems.

- Having read the information given to the simulated patient, what do you now think this station is testing?
- Make notes or discuss your thoughts with a colleague before you turn the page.

Review your approach to this station:

Tested at this station:

1. Diversity issues: communicating with a hearing-impaired patient
2. History taking skills
3. Physical examination
4. Problem-solving and diagnostic skills

Domain I – Interpersonal skills

Diversity issues: communicating with a hearing-impaired patient

Nine million people in the UK are deaf or hard of hearing. Understanding how to communicate effectively with these patients is a key skill for health-care professionals:

- The Disability Discrimination Act 1995 (DDA) gives equal access to services such as healthcare.
- Under the DDA reasonable adjustments must be made by GPs to allow equitable access to services.
- The GP curriculum points out that reasonable adjustments can be simple strategies such as remembering always to face hard of hearing or deaf patients, and to talk slowly and clearly, to allow patients to lip read.
- As you have been made aware of the patient's hearing impairment, you need to be explicit in checking understanding at regular intervals during the consultation. However, it is important to do this in an appropriate and non-patronizing manner.
- An awareness of the needs of hearing-impaired patients and taking simple steps as outlined above can help overcome communication barriers to the doctor–patient relationship.

Domain 2 – Data gathering, examination and clinical assessment skills

History taking skills

Patients often present with non-specific symptoms such as tiredness. In taking a focused history, you need to tease out relevant symptoms to help reach a working diagnosis:

- She says that she is tired and run down, can she say more about this?
- How long has she been feeling like this?
- Any other symptoms such as headaches, urinary problems, excessive thirst, bowel disturbance, abdominal pains, weight changes, fevers, cold or heat intolerance, menstrual problems, chest pain, cough or shortness of breath?
- Any visual problems or numbness, pins and needles or weakness in any of her limbs?
- It is always worth asking depression screening questions to patients who present with non-specific symptoms such as tiredness (see Examination 1: Station 1).
- Has she suffered from any other medical problems in the past?

- Does she take any medication?
- What line of work is she in? Are her symptoms affecting her work?
- Does she smoke? How much alcohol does she drink? Is there anyone at home with her?
- Are there any medical problems in her immediate family, such as diabetes or thyroid problems?
- She says that she is worried that there is something seriously wrong – does she have any thoughts about what this might be? What does she hope will happen from coming to the surgery today?

Physical examination

From the history you will hopefully have picked up that her symptoms suggest a thyroid disorder. Under the *Metabolic problems* section of the new GP curriculum, clinical examination of the neck is listed as a psychomotor skill you should be able to demonstrate. An appropriate physical examination at this station should therefore include the neck, together with looking for systemic features of thyroid disease:

- Before any physical examination, explain to the patient what will be involved and gain verbal consent to proceed.
- Brief systemic thyroid examination could include:
  ○ Pulse – can be slow and of low volume in hypothyroidism or raised in hyperthyroidism.
  ○ Is there a tremor? – Ask the patient to stretch their arms out in front of them and splay their fingers. Can be present in hyperthyroidism.
  ○ Loss of the outer third of eyebrows and dry, brittle hair can be present in hypothyroid disease.
  ○ Eyes – look for exophthalmos (protruding appearance) and lid lag. Thyroid eye disease is usually associated with Graves' disease but can occur in chronic autoimmune thyroiditis.
  ○ Reflexes – may be slow relaxing in hypothyroidism or brisk in hyperthyroidism.
- Examination of the neck:
  ○ Inspection – any scars? Any thyroid swelling (goitre) visible?
  ○ If you see a swelling ask the patient to take a sip of water – a goitre will rise on swallowing.
  ○ Palpation – best done from behind the patient. Feel for lymph nodes and assess the thyroid gland itself. Is it enlarged? Tender? What is its consistency?
  ○ Percussion – over the manubrium (upper part of the sternum). If dull this may signify a retrosternal goitre.
  ○ Auscultation – listening for bruits over the gland.

In the CSA, you will be handed a piece of paper if there are any abnormal findings from your examination.

Abnormal findings in this case include a pulse of 56 and a large diffuse goitre.

Domain 3 – Clinical management skills

Problem-solving and diagnostic skills

The GP curriculum states that thyroid disorders are very common and have an enormous impact on quality of life, but that the diagnosis is often missed. Patients who present with tiredness should always alert you to the possibility of thyroid disease:

- This patient gives a clear history suggesting hypothyroidism.
- Examination findings of bradycardia with a diffuse goitre are also consistent with this diagnosis (see Knowledge-base).
- You need to confirm the diagnosis with blood tests, namely thyroid function tests (see Knowledge-base). You should also check glucose, lipid profile, FBC and U&Es.
- You should discuss the probable diagnosis with the patient and explain the need for confirmatory blood tests. Is she happy to have the tests?
- When the patient came into the consultation room she said that she was concerned there was something 'seriously wrong'. You need to reassure her that there are no worrying findings and that, if an underactive thyroid is confirmed, the condition is very common and easily treated with tablets.
- Ask her to return after she has had the blood tests to discuss the results.
- Is she happy with the explanation and plan, and does she have any questions?

Knowledge-base – Hypothyroidism

References – NHS Clinical Knowledge Summaries.

Hypothyroidism	• Undersecretion of thyroid hormone • Overt hypothyroidism = TSH raised with low free T_4 level • Subclinical hypothyroidism = TSH raised with normal free T_4 level
Causes	• Iodine deficiency (rare in UK) • Autoimmune hypothyroidism (Hashimoto's thyroiditis = autoimmune thyroiditis and goitre) • Post thyroid surgery or radioactive iodine treatment for hyperthyroidism • Drug side effects – e.g. amiodarone and lithium • Secondary to pituitary or hypothalamic disease • Congenital hypothyroidism
How common?	Approximately 1 in 50 women and 1 in 1000 men develop hypothyroidism during their lifetime
Symptoms and signs	• Generalized tiredness and lethargy, slowing down of mental processes • Cold intolerance • Weight gain • Constipation • Absent, irregular or heavy periods • Dry skin, hair loss and hoarse or deep voice • Carpel tunnel syndrome • Low mood and reduced libido • Diffuse goitre • Myxoedema – non-pitting oedema • Slowly relaxing tendon reflexes • Bradycardia • Hypercholesterolaemia • Galactorrhoea – secondary to increased prolactin levels
Investigations	Thyroid function tests: TSH, T_4, free T_4, T_3 and thyroid antibodies
Treatment	• Levothyroxine daily • Start at 50–100 µg OD (25 µg if elderly or ischaemic heart disease) • Monitor TFTs and titrate up every 2–3 months if required
Drug interactions	• Carbamazepine, phenytoin and rifampicin accelerate the metabolism of levothyroxine • Levothyroxine enhances the anticoagulation effects of warfarin • Cimetidine and oral iron reduce absorption of levothyroxine
Free prescriptions	Those receiving levothyroxine are entitled to free prescriptions for all their medicines

- Refer patients with hypothyroidism to an endocrinologist if they are under 16 years old, pregnant or postpartum, have ischaemic heart disease, are taking amiodarone or lithium, or if you suspect pituitary or hypothalamic disease.

Take home messages

- For patients with hearing impairment, making small adjustments within the consultation can significantly improve doctor–patient communication.
- Physical examination skills must be demonstrated by candidates in the CSA.
- The GP curriculum makes clear that management of thyroid disease in primary care is a key competence for general practice.

Ideas for further revision

Practise mock consultations with a colleague where you imagine that they need to lip read what you say. Try to modify the consultation and any examination to allow adequate doctor–patient communication.

Further reading

British Deaf Association. www.britishdeafassociation.org.uk.

British Thyroid Foundation. www.btf-thyroid.org.

NHS National Library for Health Clinical Knowledge Summaries – hypothyroidism. www.cks.library.nhs.uk/clinical_knowledge.

Pop VJ. Thyroid disorders. In: Jones R, Britten N, Culpepper L, et al. (eds) *Oxford Textbook of Primary Medical Care*. Oxford: Oxford University Press, 2004.

Rehman HU, Bajwa TA. 10-minute consultation: Newly diagnosed hypothyroidism. *BMJ* 2004;**329**:1271. www.bmj.com.

Royal National Institute for Deaf People. www.rnid.org.uk.

Thyroid UK – information and advice for patients. www.thyroiduk.org.

Information given to candidates

The appointment has been booked by Raymond Mallory's sister – Stephanie Mallory. She wants to talk to you about Raymond, who has Down's syndrome and is a patient at your practice. Raymond's sister lives 70 miles away and is attending on her own today.

Raymond is 44 years old and lives in a residential housing project for people with mild to moderate learning disabilities. The project is staffed 24 h a day.

Raymond suffers from diabetes and heart failure, secondary to an incompetent mitral valve. His current medication is:

Spironolactone	25 mg OD	Bisoprolol	10 mg OD
Furosemide	80 mg OD	Metformin	500 mg TDS
Ramipril	5 mg BD	Gliclazide	80 mg OD

The last letter from the cardiologist from a month ago noted that Raymond's heart failure appeared to be gradually deteriorating despite treatment. His renal function is normal and his diabetes well controlled. The cardiologist is due to see him again in 1 month.

Raymond has had three admissions (all under 1 week's stay) in the last year as a result of worsening breathlessness secondary to heart failure.

On the last admission Raymond was assessed by one of the psychiatrists who judged that he had the capacity to discharge himself early, against medical advice.

Raymond has not appointed anyone to make medical decisions on his behalf (Lasting Powers of Attorney).

As Stephanie Mallory enters the room she says, "Doctor, I want to talk to you about Raymond. He's been so unwell over the last year, the family doesn't think he should go into hospital again if his breathing gets bad."

- What do you think this station is testing?
- Make notes or discuss your thoughts with a colleague before you read on.

Plan your approach to this station:

Information given to simulated relative

Basic details – You are Stephanie Mallory, a Caucasian 50-year-old woman, and the older sister of Raymond Mallory, who is a patient at the practice. You are attending on your own today. You live 70 miles away and visit Raymond once a month for the weekend.

Appearance and behaviour – You are well presented and assertive. If the doctor does not agree to your request to keep Raymond out of hospital, without speaking to him first, then you will initially be a little shocked. However, if the doctor explains carefully why this is the case, and takes your perspective and concerns into account, then you will accept this.

History
Freely divulged to doctor – You want to talk to the doctor about your brother – Raymond – who has Down's syndrome. Raymond had an operation on one of his heart valves when he was a baby, and over the last 4 years has been suffering from 'heart failure'. He used to see the local heart specialist once every 6 months, as initially things weren't too bad. But now he's very breathless even if he potters around in the garden and his lips always have a bluish tinge. He now sees the heart doctor every 2–3 months.

Divulged to doctor if specifically asked – Raymond is now taking lots of medication, and the heart failure specialist nurse visits every 2–3 weeks to see how he is doing. His ankle swelling seems to have got worse over the last few months, even though Raymond and his carers know that he needs to be careful with how much he drinks. He still seems generally happy and his keyworker – one of the residential home staff – often takes him out on trips or to various groups. Raymond does not seem to know what the heart doctor said to him when he last saw her 1 month ago. Raymond knows that his heart is not working properly and that he has to take all his tablets to help it. You have not discussed with Raymond what he would like to happen if his breathing gets bad again. You have only discussed this with one of Raymond's three other brothers. Raymond does not know that you are coming to see the doctor today.

Ideas, concerns and expectations – You still feel a little guilty about moving so far away when your partner got a new job 4 years ago. Raymond has always disliked going into hospital. But over the last year he has become more and more distressed when he has gone in, so much so that the last time he was admitted he came home early, against medical advice. With his worsening condition, and his hatred of hospitals, you believe that he should not have to undergo this trauma again if his breathing deteriorates, and should instead be kept at home. You want the doctor to agree with you today that Raymond will stay at home if his breathing gets bad again, rather than going into hospital, and you would like this written in his notes.

First words spoken to doctor – "Doctor, I want to talk to you about Raymond. He's been so unwell over the last year, the family doesn't think he should go into hospital again if his breathing gets bad."

Past medical history – You are fit and well. Raymond suffers from 'heart failure' and diabetes.

Drug history – You do not take any medication. You know that Raymond is on lots of tablets for his heart failure and diabetes.

Social history – You live 70 miles away with your own family. You work as a primary schoolteacher.

Family history – Apart from Raymond's problems, there are no other significant medical problems in your immediate family.

- Having read the information given to the simulated relative, what do you now think this station is testing?
- Make notes or discuss your thoughts with a colleague before you turn the page.

Review your approach to this station:

Tested at this station:

1. Addressing a relative's concerns
2. History taking
3. Respecting patient autonomy
4. Negotiating with a patient's relative

Domain 1 – Interpersonal skills

Addressing a relative's concerns

This station is primarily about addressing the concerns of a patient's close relative, while respecting patient autonomy and confidentiality in negotiating a way forward. As such, your ability to relate to Raymond's sister in an empathetic and supportive way is a key skill:

- Raymond's sister is obviously concerned about her brother's wellbeing. You should acknowledge this and ask her to say more about her worries.
- She mentions him being 'so unwell' over the last year. Can she say more about this?
- Is there any particular reason why she is so worried about him going into hospital again? Did anything happen in the last few admissions which upset or concerned her?
- What sort of impact has Raymond's learning disability had on her life?
- Has it been difficult balancing her own life with helping to support Raymond?
- Has Raymond ever mentioned what he would like to happen if his health deteriorates further?
- Has she discussed this matter with anyone else?

Domain 2 – Data gathering, examination and clinical assessment skills

History taking

It would be useful to obtain further details about Raymond's health, to help inform you when negotiating a way forward with his sister:

- How is Raymond doing at the moment?
- What is he able to do? What is he not able to do? Is he getting out?
- How have things changed over the last year?
- Does Raymond understand what is happening with his heart problem?
- Is he taking his medication as prescribed?
- Has Raymond said anything that might make you think his poor health is getting him down?
- Has his behaviour changed in any way recently?

Domain 3 – Clinical management skills

Respecting patient autonomy

All adult patients have a right to respect for autonomy (self-determination):

- Under the Mental Capacity Act 2005 for England and Wales, adult patients are presumed to have the capacity to make decisions for themselves, unless proven otherwise (see Examination 2: Station 1).
- Stephanie Mallory is asking you to make an advance decision regarding withholding care from Raymond, should his condition deteriorate. You cannot agree to this request without consulting Raymond himself.
- Just because a patient has a learning disability does not mean that they are incapable of making decisions regarding their medical care. Indeed, Raymond was judged to have the capacity to make the decision to discharge himself during his last admission.
- Although Stephanie believes she has Raymond's best interests at heart, and is a close relative, she has no legal right to determine Raymond's medical treatment.
- Nonetheless, it is good practice to involve relatives in key decisions, with the patient's consent.
- Given Raymond's gradual deterioration, it would be good practice to discuss with him his wishes should he become very ill.

Negotiating with a patient's relative

Although you are not able to agree to Stephanie's request that you keep Raymond at home if he becomes unwell again, you should focus on positive ways forward, emphasizing the need to involve Raymond at all stages:

- You need sensitively to explain that it is important to involve Raymond in any decisions about his future care.
- You could suggest that Stephanie first discusses the issue with Raymond – what does he want to happen if he becomes ill again? What did he think about being in hospital?
- You could also suggest that Stephanie speak with Raymond's other brothers – what are their thoughts on the matter?
- Involving his keyworker might also be useful – Stephanie could ask her whether Raymond has ever talked about his wishes if he becomes ill again.
- You could offer to see Raymond to discuss things further. If Raymond is happy, then you could see them both together. Also, you could ask the heart failure nurse specialist to attend too, if Raymond is OK with this.
- Raymond and his sister may also find it helpful to discuss the issue with his cardiologist at the next appointment.
- You need to be careful not to breach patient confidentiality when negotiating how best to proceed.

Knowledge-base

Common and/or important conditions associated with learning disabilities

Reference – GP curriculum statement 14, including appendix 1.

- *Epilepsy* – increased incidence and complexity with severity of learning disability.
- *Sensory impairments* – hearing and vision, earwax.
- *Obesity* – predisposes to other medical problems.
- *Gastrointestinal* – swallowing problems, reflux oesophagitis, *Helicobacter pylori* infection, constipation, gastric carcinoma.
- *Respiratory problems* – chest infections, aspiration pneumonia.
- *Cerebral palsy* – especially with severe learning disability.
- *Orthopaedic problems* – joint contractures, osteoporosis.
- *Dermatological problems.*
- *Psychiatric problems* – emotional and behavioural disorders, sexual and physical abuse, schizophrenia, bipolar affective disorder, Alzheimer's disease in Down's syndrome.

Diagnostic overshadowing

Reference – Newcastle University reference in Further reading.

The GP curriculum warns against 'diagnostic overshadowing', which is when the presenting complaint of a patient with a learning disability is put down to their learning disability, rather than health professionals looking for another cause.

It suggests that if a patient with a learning disability presents with a new behaviour, or the existing ones escalate, you should not dismiss these symptoms as simply due to their learning disability but consider physical, psychiatric and social causes:

- *Physical and psychiatric causes* – see above.
- *Social causes* – change in carers, bereavement, abuse.

Take home messages

- Patients with learning disabilities have the same right to respect for patient autonomy as other patients.
- Make sure you involve patients with learning disabilities as fully as possible in decisions about their care.
- When those close to patients consult you about their relative's/ spouse's care, you need to address their concerns in an empathic and supportive way.

Ideas for further revision

Some CSA stations will primarily be concerned with issues around professionalism and ethics. These topics are specifically covered in the GP curriculum. You should be familiar with the curriculum document, and also with key professional guidelines, including those related to confidentiality and consent.

Further reading

Department of Health. *Valuing People: A New Strategy for Learning Disability for the 21st Century.* London: DoH, 2001. Summary: www.niace.org.uk/organisation/Advocacy/ValuingPeople/Valuing%20People%20Summary.pdf.

General Medical Council. *Seeking Patients' Consent: The Ethical Considerations.* London: GMC, 1998. www.gmc-uk.org/guidance/current/library/consent.asp. (Note: this guidance is currently under review.)

General Medical Council. *Confidentiality: Protecting and Providing Information.* London: GMC, 2004. www.gmc-uk.org/guidance/current/library/confidentiality.asp.

Mencap. *'Treat me Right' Better Healthcare for People with a Learning Disability.* London: Mencap, 2004. www.mencap.org.uk/treatmeright.

Newcastle University. *The Role of Doctors in Treating People with Learning Disability* (part of which forms appendix 1 of RCGP curriculum statement 3.3). www.ncl.ac.uk/nnp/teaching/disorders/learning/ld_role.html.

NHS National Library for Health Clinical Knowledge Summaries – Down's Syndrome. www.cks.library.nhs.uk/clinical_knowledge.

RCGP curriculum statement 14 – Care of People with Learning Disabilities and RCGP curriculum statement 3.3 – Clinical Ethics and Values-based Practice. www.rcgp.org.uk.

Information given to candidates

> Margaret Stewart is a 58-year-old female patient who rarely comes to the surgery.
>
> She has been taking ramipril 2.5 mg for hypertension for 2 years and her blood pressure is well controlled on medication.

As she enters the consultation room the patient says, "This ringing in my ears is really getting me down doctor."

- What do you think this station is testing?
- Make notes or discuss your thoughts with a colleague before you read on.

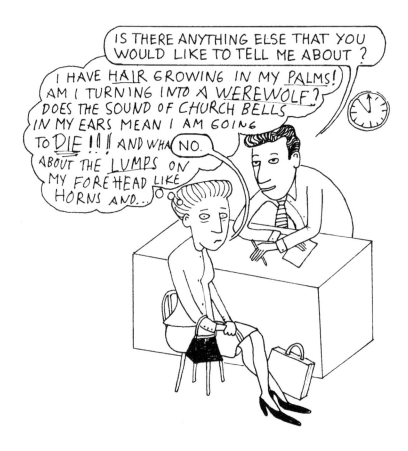

Plan your approach to this station:

Information given to simulated patient

Basic details – You are Margaret Stewart, a Caucasian, divorced, 58-year-old social worker.

Appearance and behaviour – You are articulate and well-presented, with good eye contact throughout the consultation.

History
Freely divulged to doctor – You noticed a ringing sound in both ears about 3 months ago. It came on gradually over a few weeks. It has not really changed since then. It is not something you have ever had before and it is now interfering with your life and making you frustrated. You have not mentioned this to anyone else. You put off coming down to the surgery as you 'don't like to bother' the doctor and thought that it would probably just go away on its own.

Divulged to doctor if specifically asked – The ringing noise worries you, and the more you worry the more you focus on the noise. Your house is quiet at night and this is when you feel the ringing is loudest. Your sleep has been disturbed over the last 2 months as you find yourself thinking about the ringing when you are trying to get off to sleep. You consider yourself 'a bit of a worrier'. You did not want to trouble other people, so you have not discussed this with your daughter or friends. You have never had your ears syringed for wax, and cannot remember the last time you even had an ear infection. Your hearing does not seem to be any worse than normal. You are eating well, you get pleasure from seeing your family, and enjoy dealing with clients at work, although the management side is quite stressful. You have not had any ear pain or discharge. You have not noticed any weakness in your facial muscles, or any other symptoms in the rest of your body. You have not felt dizzy or noticed a problem with your balance. Although you have got frustrated with the ringing, you do not think you are depressed. You have not banged your head recently and have not been suffering from a cold.

Ideas, concerns and expectations – You were very close to your grandfather when you were younger. You remember that he always complained about his ears. You were 8 when your mother told you that he had died from a brain tumour, and since the problem with your ears started you have been worried that the same thing might be happening to you. You are keen for the doctor to explain to you what is going on and ideally reassure you that it is not anything serious. You will be happy to try any self-help measures that the doctor suggests.

First words spoken to doctor – "This ringing in my ears is really getting me down doctor."

Past medical history – Two years ago you were found to have high blood pressure. You spent a few months trying to bring the blood pressure down by adopting a healthier lifestyle, but this did not seem to work so you started taking tablets. The medication appears to have worked as the nurse always says that things are fine at your 6-monthly check-ups. Apart from minor illnesses you have otherwise been fit and well. You have never suffered from depression.

Drug history – You take a tablet – ramipril 2.5 mg once a day – for high blood pressure. You are not allergic to any medication.

Social history – You are a full-time social worker. The job has been getting more and more stressful over recent years, particularly since you were promoted to team leader 3 years ago. You split up with your husband 10 years ago and now live on your own. You have one adult daughter who lives nearby and has her own family – a partner and two boys. You have never smoked. You drink less than a bottle of wine a week.

Family history – There are no major health problems in your immediate family.

- Having read the information given to the simulated patient, what do you now think this station is testing?
- Make notes or discuss your thoughts with a colleague before you turn the page.

Review approach to this station:

Tested at this station:

1. Identifying a hidden agenda
2. History taking skills
3. Physical examination
4. Management of common medical conditions presenting in primary care

Domain 1 – Interpersonal skills

Identifying a hidden agenda

This patient is concerned that she has a brain tumour. However, you are unlikely to uncover this unless you elicit her thoughts about what happened to her grandfather:

- In the CSA be alert to cues – either verbal or non-verbal – from the patient.
- Just a simple, 'Have you any concerns?' may not be enough to elicit a patient's deepest fears.
- Use good listening skills, go at the patient's pace and be empathic. The patient will be more likely to open up if you adopt such an approach.
- When you are trying to identify a patient's ideas, concerns and expectations, it is often useful to ask if any friends or family members have experienced similar symptoms. What happened to them? Does the patient think the same might happen to her?
- If you are half-way through a CSA station but get the sense that you are missing some key element to the consultation, then it is worth revisiting the patient's ideas, concerns and expectations. At this stage, questions such as, *"Is there anything else you would like to tell me?"* can prove fruitful.

Domain 2 – Data gathering, examination and clinical assessment skills

History taking skills

Although the causes of tinnitus are usually benign, it is important to take a thorough history to try and exclude serious causes (see Knowledge-base), and to assess the impact on the patient's life:

- Start with open questions – Can she say more about the ringing in her ears? In what way is it getting her down? How is she coping with the noise? What are her thoughts about what is going on? What was she hoping would happen from coming to the surgery today?
- More specific questions that you could ask include:
  - Is there ringing in both ears or just one?
  - Is it present all the time, or does it come and go?
  - How long has she noticed the ringing?
  - What makes it better? What makes it worse?
  - Any associated symptoms with the ringing?
  - How intrusive does she find the noise? Does it affect her sleep?
  - Does it stop her doing things?

○ Any previous ear problems? How is her hearing?
○ What medication has she taken over the last 6 months?
○ Any previous exposure to high levels of noise? What is her job?
○ How are things at home? Any major life events recently?
○ Has she banged her head recently?

Physical examination

At this station you would be expected to examine the patient's ears and test her hearing – see Examination 1: Station 6. You should also examine her cranial nerves – particularly V and VII (see Further reading).

You will be told that all the examinations are normal.

Domain 3 – Clinical management skills

Management of common medical conditions presenting in primary care

The patient is experiencing bilateral tinnitus (the perception of noise with no external stimulus):

- You should reassure her that although the noise can be distressing, it is common and there are a number of ways to help with the condition.
- Explicitly address her fear about it being cancer and explain that none of the symptoms or signs suggests anything serious.
- You could suggest organizing some simple blood tests – FBC, U&Es and TFTs – to ensure that you are not missing any general health problem. What does the patient think about this?
- The GP curriculum states that with tinnitus you should try and empower patients to adopt self-treatment and coping strategies. Self-help advice which you could discuss with the patient includes:
  ○ General sleep hygiene measures – e.g. avoiding caffeine in the evening, trying to do some exercise during the day, and winding down before bedtime.
  ○ Relaxation techniques – going to a local class or buying a tape.
  ○ Background noise – this will help focus the brain away from the tinnitus (e.g. radio hiss, leaving windows open, using a fan).
  ○ Joining a local self-help group for further advice and support – such as those run by the British Tinnitus Association (see Further reading).
- Ask to see the patient again for a review in a month's time – or sooner if she has any concerns or new symptoms. Explain that if the tinnitus continues to cause problems despite self-help measures, then there is the option of referral for tinnitus retraining therapy – which includes cognitive behaviour therapy (CBT) and sound therapy (e.g. white noise generators or hearing aids to increase background noise).
- Referral to an ENT specialist would also be an option if the ringing continued to be intrusive.

Knowledge-base – Tinnitus

References – NHS Clinical Knowledge Summaries, BMJ Tinnitus article – see Further reading.

	Associated with tinnitus
More commonly	• Damage to the cochlear or other inner ear apparatus • Presbyacusis – natural hearing loss in the elderly • Long term exposure to excessive noise – e.g. occupational hazard, non-use of ear protectors • Middle ear infections • Perforated tympanic membrane • Ménière's disease • Otosclerosis • Anaemia • Excessive wax
Less commonly	• Exposure to sudden or very loud noise – e.g. gunfire, explosion • Head injury • Impacted wisdom teeth • Medication – e.g. diuretics, tricyclics, quinine, aminoglycosides, aspirin, NSAIDs • Solvent or alcohol misuse • High blood pressure • Hyperthyroidism
Rarely	• Acoustic neuroma

Refer to a specialist if:

- Objective tinnitus (can be heard by an observer)
- Pulsatile tinnitus (unless due to an acute inflammatory ear infection)
- Unilateral tinnitus without an obvious cause (such as exposure to a recent loud noise on that side)
- Persistent intrusive tinnitus
- Associated deafness.

Take home messages

- If you are patient-centred during consultations, then the patient's agenda is more likely to be revealed.
- You need to feel confident in the management of common conditions presenting in primary care.
- Always remember to 'safety net' with appropriate follow-up or explicit instructions on when patients should re-present.

Ideas for further revision

The CSA uses a series of blueprints to ensure that for each 13-station examination there is a range of complexity in the cases. There will also be a balance to the nature of cases (e.g. acute problems, chronic disease management, diversity and ethical issues, etc). Furthermore, each CSA will contain stations covering a variety of systems (e.g. ENT, cardiovascular, respiratory, women's health, etc). Try to ensure your revision takes account of all these dimensions, and use the GP curriculum to identify gaps in your knowledge.

Further reading

British Tinnitus Association – information sheets for patients and health professionals. www.tinnitus.org.uk.

ENT UK – includes patient information on a range of ENT conditions. www. entuk.org.

Hannan SA, Sami F, Wareing MJ. 10-minute consultation – tinnitus. *BMJ* 2005;**330**:237. www.bmj.com.

NHS National Library for Health Clinical Knowledge Summaries – tinnitus. www.cks.library.nhs.uk/clinical_knowledge.

RCGP curriculum statement 15.4 – Clinical Management: ENT and facial problems. www.rcgp.org.uk.

Thomas J, Monaghan T. *Oxford Handbook of Clinical Examination and Practical Skills*. Oxford: Oxford University Press, 2007.

Examination 2: Station 5

Information given to candidates

> Angus Henderson is a 32-year-old patient who has been registered with the practice for 8 years but who has only attended on three occasions – once for a life insurance medical check and twice for minor, self-limiting illnesses.

As the patient enters the room he says, "I'm sorry to waste your time doctor but my wife made me come down. Things have been a bit blurry in my right eye – just the central bit – for a few weeks, but it's back to normal now and I'm sure it's nothing to worry about. I just need to get my eyes checked at the optician, don't you think?"

- What do you think this station is testing?
- Make notes or discuss your thoughts with a colleague before you read on.

Plan your approach to this station:

Information given to simulated patient

Basic details – You are Angus Henderson, a Caucasian 32-year-old bus driver.

Appearance and behaviour – You come across as being dismissive that there might be anything seriously wrong. Deep down you are in fact worried, but you are overcompensating for this by your unconcerned, nonchalant attitude with the doctor today. You will try and cajole the doctor into agreeing with you that all is well. If the doctor is caring and empathetic, but clear in explaining that your symptoms cannot be so easily dismissed, then you will be inclined to disclose your true concerns and ask the doctor directly if you could have multiple sclerosis.

History

Freely divulged to doctor – Four weeks ago you noticed a problem with the vision in your right eye. If you covered up your left eye, then there seemed to be a central patch that was very blurred. Your left eye was fine, and things cleared up completely within 3 weeks. You have had floaters in both eyes in the past and so dismissed it as probably being due to a large floater, although you have never had a floater that big and previously floaters have not made your vision blurred. Your vision is back to normal now.

Divulged to doctor if specifically asked – Your right eye was painful if you moved it during the time when your vision was affected. You nearly had an accident while driving your bus at work a couple of weeks ago when the car in front braked suddenly just as you were scratching your left eyelid. You did not see the car properly until you opened your left eye, due to the blurred vision. You have not had any headaches or any weakness in your limbs or face. If the doctor specifically asks about times in the past when you may have had sensory symptoms, you will remember that a couple of years ago you had tingling sensations and some numbness in the toes of your left foot for about a week, which you put down to a new pair of tight shoes. You have had no such symptoms since then. Your speech has been normal. You have not had any bladder or bowel problems.

Ideas, concerns and expectations – You think of yourself as extremely fit and healthy – it has been years since you came to see the doctor and you have never been in hospital. Deep down you are concerned that you are suffering from something serious – you had heard about multiple sclerosis on the radio and know that it can start with eye problems. You have been coping with these fears by convincing yourself that there is nothing really to worry about as things have resolved completely and you are in such good health generally. You have not discussed your fears with your wife, but she made you book an appointment at the surgery as she knew about the blurred vision and insisted you should get things checked out. You want the doctor to go along with your expressed view that this is nothing serious, as this will allay your fears. To this end you will underplay the visual problem you have had, unless the doctor asks specific questions about your symptoms.

First words spoken to doctor – "I'm sorry to waste your time doctor but my wife made me come down. Things have been a bit blurry in my right eye – just the central bit – for a few weeks, but it's back to normal now and I'm sure it's nothing to worry about. I just need to get my eyes checked at the optician, don't you think?"

Past medical history – Apart from the tingling sensation and numbness in your toes a couple of years ago, you are fit and well. You have only been to the doctor's three times in the last 8 years – once for a life insurance medical and twice for coughs and colds.

Drug history – You do not take any regular medication and you have no drug allergies.

Social history – You are married with three young children. You go running three or four times a week. You drink the odd pint of beer at the weekend, unless you are working. You have never smoked.

Family history – There is no history of any of your family having eye or major health problems.

- Having read the information given to the simulated patient, what do you now think this station is testing?
- Make notes or discuss your thoughts with a colleague before you turn the page.

Review your approach to this station:

Tested at this station:

1. Dealing with a dismissive patient
2. History taking skills
3. Reaching a shared management plan

Domain 1 – Interpersonal skills

Dealing with a dismissive patient

This patient has significant recent symptoms that he is trying to trivialize, in an attempt to allay his fears that there may be something seriously wrong:

- This patient wants you to agree with him that the recent episode of blurred vision is nothing to worry about. He will try and play down the extent and severity of his symptoms and encourage you to confirm that a visit to the optician is all that is required.
- In one sense he is superficially in denial about his symptoms. Denial can be a powerful coping mechanism when patients are confronted with the potentially serious implications of certain symptoms or diagnoses. However, on another level he is aware of and frightened by the implications of his blurred vision, although he has tried to suppress these concerns, even to himself.
- Initially the patient will be quite manipulative in trying to get you to agree that this is only a minor problem and that all is well. In response, you need to be clear that you do not think this is something that can so readily be dismissed.
- The key here is to be able to feel comfortable in disagreeing with the patient – albeit in a professional and non-confrontational manner. Responses such as – *"Well, I'm not so sure"* or *"I can see why you might believe that but I don't think we can just dismiss your symptoms without further investigations"*, may be useful.
- You will have to employ all your interpersonal skills to try and tease out his true concerns. You need to demonstrate to him through active listening, non-verbal communication and a caring, empathic approach that you are a doctor he can open up to.
- Probing his thoughts about what has happened may also help – Why does he think the blurred vision is a minor problem? Did he ever think this might be something more serious? What does he think caused the symptoms?

Domain 2 – Data gathering, examination and clinical assessment skills

History taking skills

The patient has presented with a worrying neurological symptom, albeit one that appears to have resolved. This case tests your ability to take a detailed history to try and uncover whether the patient has experienced any other neurological deficits in the past, to help narrow down the differential diagnoses:

- He mentions having some blurred vision in his right eye, can he say more about this?
- When did he first notice this? What was it like?
- Did he have any other eye symptoms, such as pain or double vision?
- Was his eye red and inflamed?
- What has his left eye been like?
- How and when did his symptoms resolve?
- Has anything like this ever happened before?
- Does he suffer from headaches?
- Any weakness, numbness or odd sensations in his face or any of his limbs? Looking back can he think of any previous episodes when he may have had funny sensations, numbness or weakness?
- Has he been affected by problems with his balance or dizziness recently or in the past?
- Any difficulty with swallowing or speech? Any memory problems?
- Any bowel, bladder or erectile problems?
- Were his symptoms worse when it was hot or if he had been exercising?
- Does he have any previous medical problems? Any regular medication?
- Does he smoke? How much alcohol does he drink?
- How has his general health been? Any fatigue or low mood?
- What job does he do?
- How did his blurred vision affect his life – at home and at work?

Physical examination

This is a fairly full station, with candidates having to deal with the patient's dismissive attitude, take a detailed history and address fitness to drive issues, all in 10 min. Given his presenting complaint, you should say that you would like to perform a full neurological examination and check his blood pressure. However, you will not be required actually to perform the examinations but will be told:

There is pallor of the right optic disc on fundoscopy. All other findings on examination of the cranial and peripheral nervous system, including visual acuity and visual fields, are normal. Blood pressure today is 128/82.

Domain 3 – Clinical management skills

Reaching a shared management plan

Initially there may be discordance between the patient's dismissive attitude and your concerns. But if you have managed to find out his deep-seated worries, then you will be in a better position to negotiate a management plan acceptable to both of you:

- His recent visual symptoms and examination findings are consistent with a diagnosis of optic neuritis, which is associated with multiple sclerosis.
- He has also experienced an episode of tingling sensations and numbness in the toes of his left foot a couple of years ago, although this could have been due to his footwear.

- Even though you may suspect a serious neurological condition, such as multiple sclerosis, from the history, it would be premature to mention a specific diagnosis to the patient at this stage. Doing so would have significant implications for the patient and you should wait for specialist input and further assessment.
- However, if he asks you directly if it could be multiple sclerosis, then you would have to reply honestly and say that it is one possibility, although you should share your uncertainty with him at this stage.
- Although multiple sclerosis is still a clinical diagnosis based on two episodes involving at least two parts of the central nervous system separated in time, the more recent McDonald criteria (see Further reading) allows earlier diagnosis, in some cases, by incorporating imaging and laboratory tests. This has the potential to facilitate earlier decisions on treatment options.
- Hence if you suspect multiple sclerosis, you should be looking to refer to a neurologist without delay.
- How does the patient feel about being referred to see a specialist?
- Does he understand that it is currently unclear what caused his visual problems but that it is important to look into this further? What are his thoughts about this?
- In the meantime you could suggest some simple screening blood tests – e.g. FBC, U&Es, glucose, B_{12} and folate. Is he OK with having these?
- You could advise the patient that the specialist might decide to organize a scan – an MRI – and describe what that would be like for the patient – e.g. *"like going into a long doughnut which makes funny noises, for about 15 min"*. Explain that the specialist may also want to take a sample of fluid from his spine together with further eye tests.
- Driver and Vehicle Licensing Agency (DVLA) issues – although the patient's visual deficit seems to have resolved, this has only been grossly tested by you today and needs further assessment. The patient has recently nearly had an accident and, given that he drives a bus and is responsible for the safety of his passengers, you should advise him to refrain from driving until he sees the neurologist. If a diagnosis of multiple sclerosis is subsequently made, then he would need to inform the DVLA, which would then decide if he is medically fit to drive.
- Refraining from driving has major implications for this patient and you should explore his thoughts and feelings about this measure.

Knowledge-base – Fitness to drive

Reference – DVLA guidance – see Further reading.

		Group 1 – includes car and motor cycles	Group 2 – includes buses and large lorries
Neurological	Epilepsy	1 year off driving after first seizure. If no further attacks, can resume after medical review. Special consideration if non-recurring provoking cause identified	10 years off driving after first seizure
	TIA and stroke	Must not drive for at least 1 month. If recovery is satisfactory after a month, then can resume driving	Licence revoked for at least 1 year. Can be considered for review thereafter if full and complete recovery
	Multiple sclerosis	Notify DVLA when a clear diagnosis is made. Impairments are variable so assessments on an individual basis. Particular attention to cognitive and visual deficits	Licence revoked if condition is progressive or disabling
Vision	Acuity	Must be able to read a number plate at a distance of 20 m	New applicants are barred if corrected visual acuity is worse than 6/9 in the better eye or 6/12 in the other eye. The uncorrected acuity in each eye must be at least 3/60
CVS	Angina	Stop driving if symptoms occur at rest or at the wheel	Licence revoked if continuing symptoms
	Myocardial infarction	Stop driving for at least 1 month	Stop driving for at least 6 weeks. Review after 6 weeks
	Hypertension	Driving may continue unless treatment causes unacceptable side effects	Disqualified from driving if resting BP consistently > 180/100 (either figure)
	Arrhythmias	Stop driving if the arrhythmia is likely to cause incapacity	Licence revoked until controlled for 3 months. Medical review includes requirement of LV ejection fraction > 0.4

		Group 1 – includes car and motor cycles	Group 2 – includes buses and large lorries
Diabetes Mellitus	Diet or tablet controlled	No restrictions unless sequelae develop – e.g. diabetic eye disease affecting vision	As for Group 1
	Controlled by insulin	Must recognize warning symptoms of hypoglycaemia and meet required visual standards. 1-, 2- or 3-year licence	From 1/4/91 new applicants are barred. Drivers licensed before 1/4/91 dealt with individually
Psychiatric disorders	Acute psychotic disorder	Driving must cease during the acute illness. Re-licensing can be considered when well for at least 3 months, compliant with treatment and favourable specialist report	Driving must cease pending a medical enquiry. Normally required to be well and stable for 3 years before re-licencing considered
	Dementia	Very difficult to assess. In early dementia when sufficient skills are retained and progression is slow, a licence may be issued subject to annual review	Licence revoked
Respiratory and sleep disorders	COPD and asthma	DVLA need not be notified unless attacks are associated with disabling giddiness, fainting or loss of consciousness	As for Group 1
	Obstructive sleep apnoea	Stop driving until satisfactory control of symptoms, confirmed by a medical review	Stop driving until satisfactory control of symptoms and ongoing compliance with treatment, confirmed by specialist

Take home messages

- Patients who appear dismissive about potentially serious symptoms may be using denial as a coping mechanism.
- Explore their health beliefs thoroughly but make clear that you do not agree that their symptoms can be so readily dismissed.
- You have a responsibility to advise patients to refrain from driving and contact the DVLA if you believe that their medical condition places them or others at risk.

Ideas for further revision

The GP curriculum states that one of the psychomotor skills you must be able to demonstrate is competence in performing a full neurological examination. Although not required at this station, this can be readily tested in the CSA, so practise with colleagues until you feel confident in your ability to perform a slick neurological examination.

Further reading

Carter T. *Fitness to Drive – A Guide for Health Professionals*. London: RSM Press, 2006.

Driver and Vehicle Licensing Agency. For Medical Practitioners: At a Glance Guide to the Current Medical Standards of Fitness to Drive. Swansea: DVLA, February 2007. www.dvla.gov.uk/medical/ataglance.aspx.

General Medical Council. *GMC Guidance – Confidentiality: Protecting and Providing Information. Frequently Asked Questions: Patients driving/ DVLA, question 17*. April 2004. www.gmc-uk.org/guidance/current/library/ confidentiality_faq.asp#q17.

Murray TJ. Diagnosis and treatment of multiple sclerosis. *BMJ* 2006;**332**:525–527. www.bmj.com. (Includes on-line summary of McDonald diagnostic criteria.)

Multiple Sclerosis Society UK – information for patients and professionals. www.mssociety.org.uk.

O'Brien MD. Taking a neurological history. *Medicine* 2004;**32**:1–6.

Examination 2: Station 6

Information given to candidates

Candidates note: The setting for this station is an **out-of-hours home visit**.

You are working a Saturday morning session for the local out-of-hours provider.

Your first call of the day is a home visit to see Ben Wayne, a 74-year-old patient at a neighbouring practice to your own.

You do not have access to his GP medical records.

The information provided by the out-of-hours triage service states:

Patient	Ben Wayne
Age	74 years old
Problem	Patient describes chest pain at approximately 2am last night. Not sure how long it lasted. Associated nausea. Patient thought it was indigestion. Not relieved by antacids. Did not radiate to arms or neck. No shortness of breath. Patient says he feels fine now.
Past history	No history of heart problems. Has had 'camera test of stomach' due to indigestion last year.
Medication	Lansoprazole 15 mg OD
Management	Patient advised to call 999 and go straight to hospital for investigation and treatment. Patient refused admission, stating he is now well and just wants 'checking over'. Agreed to home visit.

The first words from the patient as you enter his house are, "I'm sorry about all the fuss, doctor. I know they wanted me to go to hospital but I'm feeling fine now and there's no way I'm going to miss seeing my new granddaughter."

- What do you think this station is testing?
- Make notes or discuss your thoughts with a colleague before you read on.

Plan your approach to this station:

Information given to simulated patient

Basic details – You are Ben Wayne, a Caucasian 74-year-old retired plumber.

Appearance and behaviour – You are a little flustered at the events of last night together with your planned trip by train to see your new granddaughter.

History

Freely divulged to doctor – You woke up at 2am earlier today with chest pain. The pain was constant and lasted about 45 min. Initially you thought it was indigestion, but it did not go away or change when you sat up or moved around. You had a glass of water and some paracetamol, but nothing seemed to make any difference to the pain. You started to get worried when the pain was still there after half an hour. By then you thought that it might be a heart problem, but now you think it was probably due to stress.

Divulged to doctor if specifically asked – The chest pain felt like severe heavy pressure over the middle of your chest. You felt nauseous and short of breath with the pain. The pain did not radiate to your neck or arms, or go through to your back. You have never experienced a pain like this before. The pain was not worse as you breathed. You have not had any pain in your calves or any leg swelling. You do not have a cough. You felt fit and well until last night. You did not experience any heart palpitations (feeling your heart beating in your chest or a rapid heart beat). The pain gradually started to ease after about 40 min and had gone within a further 5 min. You were able to go back to sleep after another half an hour. You woke up feeling a little tired, but otherwise OK. There has been no recurrence of the pain. You do not want your daughter to know what has happened.

Ideas, concerns and expectations – You have not told your daughter what happened as you know she will tell you not to travel and you really want to see your first grandchild. You think that the pain was probably due to stress over all the travel arrangements. At one point you did think that the pain might be coming from your heart, but because it went away and you now feel absolutely fine, you do not think that it could be anything serious like a heart attack. But you thought you should speak to someone about it, so you rang your GP surgery in the morning and were transferred through to the out-of-hours service. When they said that you should dial 999 and go straight to hospital you thought they were being over-cautious. You told them that you did not think you needed to go to hospital, but agreed to a home visit from the doctor. The idea of going to hospital is also distressing as it reminds you of when your wife was very ill. You expect that once the doctor sees how well you are, they won't say that you should go straight to hospital. If the doctor does ask you to go now, you will strongly resist this request. Even if the doctor says that you may well have had a heart attack and could risk your life without immediate treatment, you will simply refuse to miss your planned trip. However, if you feel confident in the doctor's abilities then – after some discussion – you will offer to go to see your own GP on your return on Monday morning, and immediately seek help if you have any further episodes of chest pain over the weekend. You will be happy to take any medication that the doctor wants to give you now.

First words spoken to doctor – "I'm sorry about all the fuss, doctor. I know they wanted me to go to hospital but I'm feeling fine now and there's no way I'm going to miss seeing my new granddaughter."

Past medical history – As far as you know, you have never had high blood pressure or any heart problems. You suffered from quite severe indigestion last year, but after having a 'camera test' and taking some tablets to get rid of 'a bug in my stomach', you have been much better. You do not recall having had your cholesterol checked.

Drug history – You take one tablet every morning for indigestion – lansoprazole 15 mg. You have no allergies.

Social history – You live on your own. Your wife died 10 years ago from breast cancer and you are very close to your only daughter who moved last year and now lives 60 miles away. You worked as a plumber until retirement 10 years ago. You gave up smoking 2 years ago but had been a heavy smoker for 30 years (about 40 cigarettes a day). You want to cut down on fried foods and eat a healthier diet.

Family history – Your father died from a stroke aged 62 and your older brother had a heart attack aged 53.

- Having read the information given to the simulated patient, what do you now think this station is testing?
- Make notes or discuss your thoughts with a colleague before you turn the page.

Review your approach to this station:

Tested at this station:

1. Understanding the patient's perspective and respecting patient autonomy
2. History taking skills
3. Recognition and management of a potentially life-threatening condition
4. Negotiating a management plan

Domain 1 – Interpersonal skills

Understanding the patient's perspective and respecting patient autonomy

Competent, fully informed patients have a right to refuse treatment, even if this puts them at risk of serious harm. Eliciting the patient's ideas, concerns and expectations will help you understand his perspective on events:

- The GP curriculum states that GPs should be able to deal sensitively and in line with professional codes of practice with patients who may have a serious diagnosis and refuse admission.
- You need to try and find out why the patient is so reluctant to go into hospital – is it just about missing his trip to see his granddaughter or are there any other concerns? In this case, he has distressing memories associated with hospital visits when his wife was ill.
- This scenario is designed to see if you can respect patient autonomy where a competent patient refuses to comply with your request for his immediate admission to hospital.
- There is a tension between your judgement of what is in his best interests and his strongly held preference to travel to see his daughter, whatever the risks.
- Although you should be frank with the patient about the potential consequences of going against medical advice, you need to be careful not to be coercive or bullying in your approach.

Domain 2 – Data gathering, examination and clinical assessment skills

History taking skills

You may feel that from the information given by the out-of-hours triage service, this patient is unlikely to have a serious condition. However, be wary of second-hand histories – these can often change dramatically when you hear the first-hand account (as in this case):

- Any complaint of chest pain needs a thorough history to try and identify life-threatening conditions such as myocardial infarction, pulmonary embolus or dissecting aortic aneurysm.
- In an out-of-hours setting, without access to the patient's medical records, taking a careful history becomes even more important.
- You need to ask various questions about the pain itself (see Knowledgebase) as part of a comprehensive cardiovascular history, including risk factors for ischaemic heart disease (see Examination 1: Station 8).

Physical examination

Due to time constraints at this station, you will not have to examine the patient. However, you would be expected to attempt to examine him, at which point the examiner will tell you the findings – namely that cardiovascular examination is normal.

Domain 3 – Clinical management skills

Recognition and management of a potentially life-threatening condition

The GP curriculum states that GPs should be competent in the recognition and immediate management of emergencies encountered in primary care (see Knowledge-base):

- The history of what happened in the night should alert you to the strong possibility that the patient has had a myocardial infarction (MI).
- In addition, this patient has a number of risk factors for heart disease and including a family history of cardiovascular disease, 60 pack years accumulated as a smoker and a high saturated fat diet.
- If you are to pass this station, you need to make it clear that you consider this a potentially life-threatening situation requiring immediate action.
- The immediate management of a patient you suspect is having an MI is listed in the Knowledge-base.
- In this case, the management is complicated by his refusal to be admitted to hospital.
- You need to treat him – as far as he will permit – to minimize the risk of further cardiac damage.

Negotiating a management plan (overlap with Domain 1)

It is essential that you elicit the patient's ideas, concerns and expectations, to allow you to engage with him in a meaningful way and to negotiate how to proceed:

- You must not collude with the patient in downplaying the potential seriousness of the current situation.
- You need to be very clear about the fact that he may well have had a heart attack and that he needs immediate assessment in hospital.
- If he is adamant that he does not want to go to hospital, you need to ensure that he understands that this is a potentially life-threatening situation.
- Even though he feels well now, you can explain that he is at very high risk of a further episode, and without appropriate treatment, this might prove fatal.
- Would he allow you to contact his daughter, or another member of the family, to discuss what has happened?
- If he continues to refuse to go straight to hospital, even though he is aware of the risks, would he be prepared to go to his daughter's local hospital, once he has seen his granddaughter? Or agree to see his own GP as soon as he returns?
- If he has any further chest pain, your advice must be to seek immediate medical help. Will he agree to this?

- Would he allow you to give him some aspirin now, and a spray to use under his tongue if he has any further chest pain? You need to explain why these are important.

Knowledge-base

References – RCGP curriculum statement 7, appendix 3, SIGN guidelines 93, *Oxford Handbook of General Practice* – see Further reading.

'Dangerous' diagnoses	Certain conditions encountered in primary care require urgent action, including:
	• Myocardial infarction (MI)
	• Pulmonary embolus
	• Subarachnoid haemorrhage
	• Appendicitis
	• Limb ischaemia
	• Intestinal obstruction or perforation
	• Meningitis
	• Aneurysms
	• Ectopic pregnancy
	• Acute psychosis/mania
	• Visual problems that could threaten blindness:
	   ○ Retinal detachment and haemorrhage
	   ○ Temporal arteritis

Cautious approach	• If you suspect any of the diagnoses above in a primary care setting, you should arrange for the patient to be transferred to a secondary care centre, to allow a more thorough assessment • At times, you may be seen to be over-cautious, but without the ability to conduct a range of investigations and close monitoring it is difficult to exclude such life-threatening conditions in primary care
Immediate management of suspected MI	In a primary care setting – either in the surgery or on a home visit – while waiting for the ambulance to arrive: • If available, give high flow oxygen • Give aspirin 300 mg – ask the patient to chew it • Give GTN – two sprays sublingually. Repeat if necessary • Gain IV access • If available, give IV diamorphine 2.5–10 mg together with an antiemetic, e.g. metoclopramide 10 mg • If possible, have a defibrillator ready
Pain history	A useful mnemonic when obtaining a detailed history of chest – and other – pain is: **SSS, OPD, RAAT** • Site – where exactly is the pain? • Sort – what does the pain feel like – sharp, dull, tight, etc? • Severity – on a scale of 1 to 10, how bad is the pain? • Onset – when did the pain start and what was the patient doing? • Periodicity – does the pain come and go or is it constant? • Duration – how long does the pain last? • Radiation – does the pain radiate anywhere? • Alleviating or worsening factors – what makes the pain better? What makes it worse? • Associated symptoms – e.g. nausea, sweating, breathlessness • Time off work – how has the pain affected the patient's life?

Take home messages

- You need to take a detailed history for all complaints of chest pain.
- Patient autonomy must be respected in competent, fully informed patients.
- You should feel confident in the initial management of life-threatening conditions seen in primary care.

Ideas for further revision

Learning objectives in the GP curriculum – which the CSA will base scenarios around – include the immediate management of acutely ill people. In this context, the curriculum states that specific psychomotor skills that you should be able to demonstrate include:

- Cardiopulmonary resuscitation (CPR) of children and adults, including use of a defibrillator.
- Performing and interpreting an electrocardiogram.
- Using a nebulizer.
- Passing a urinary catheter.
- Controlling a haemorrhage and suturing a wound.

Although these skills may be assessed in a workplace-based setting, you could be presented in the CSA with a scenario that requires candidates – as part of the station – to demonstrate one of these skills either on a simulated patient or a manikin. Make sure that you feel confident in performing such tasks competently. You may consider that you would benefit from attending a refresher course to keep you life support skills up to date.

Further reading

Committee of General Practice Education Directors. *Out of Hours (OOH) Training for GP Registrars*. London: COGPED, 2004. www.cogped.org.uk/ document_store/1139305073itpm_out_of_hours_position_paper.doc.

NHS National Library for Health Clinical Knowledge Summaries – Angina. www.cks.library.nhs.uk/clinical_knowledge.

RCGP curriculum statement 7 – Care of acutely ill people. www.rcgp.org.uk. Also see appendix 3 reference: Medical Protection Society. *Casebook Vol. 13 No. 3*. London: Medical Protection Society, 2005.

Scottish Intercollegiate Guidelines Network (SIGN) guidelines 93. Acute coronary syndromes. February 2007. www.sign.ac.uk/pdf/sign93.pdf.

Simon C, Everitt H, Kendrick T. *Oxford Handbook of General Practice*, 2nd edn. Oxford: Oxford University Press, 2005.

Thomas J, Monaghan T. *Oxford Handbook of Clinical Examination and Practical Skills*. Oxford: Oxford University Press, 2007.

Information given to candidates

> Marcus Harrison is a 58-year-old patient who rarely comes to the surgery.
>
> His records show that he had a duodenal ulcer when he was 33 years old, for which he required surgery. He has not had any related symptoms since then.

As Marcus enters the consultation room you can see that he is not moving his right arm, but has it flexed at the elbow and held against his body.

The first words the patient says when he enters the room are, "Sorry to bother you, doctor, but my right shoulder has been giving me so much trouble. I can't sleep and driving my taxi is getting to be a real problem. I know that I shouldn't be taking the Brufen but it's the only thing that helps the pain. It's really starting to get me down."

- What do you think this station is testing?
- Make notes or discuss your thoughts with a colleague before you read on.

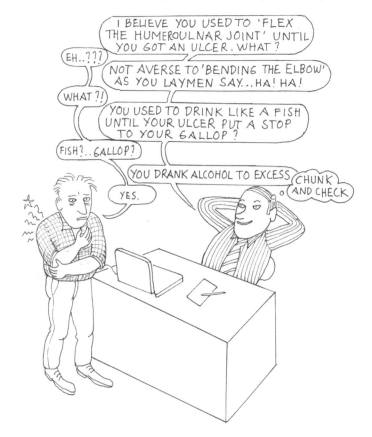

Plan your approach to this station:

Information given to simulated patient

Basic details – You are Marcus Harrison, a Caucasian 58-year-old taxi driver.

Appearance and behaviour – When you enter the consulting room you are holding your right arm against your body, with it bent at the elbow. If the doctor examines your shoulder there are no specific tender points but it feels generally sore. You find it painful to move your right arm at the shoulder in any direction, whether against resistance or not (i.e. forwards, backwards, outwards or twisting the arm inwards or outwards), but you are able to do so by about 30° in all directions (i.e. about a third of the way between having your arm by your side and having your elbow at the same height as your shoulder). The only exception to this is twisting or rotating the shoulder outwards – this is particularly painful and you cannot really manage this at all, as the pain is so bad. You will not be able to put your right hand behind your head or place your right hand in the small of your back, if asked to do so by the doctor. Your left shoulder is fine.

History
Freely divulged to doctor – You do not normally come to the doctor's but your right shoulder has been giving you problems for the last 4 weeks. It started off as a general ache with the joint feeling stiff. It has become increasingly painful with restricted movement. You have been finding it hard to sleep as the pain wakes you up and is particularly bad if you lie on your right side. With the pain and not sleeping, things are really getting you down.

Divulged to doctor if specifically asked – You do not remember injuring or straining your shoulder. You feel the pain most in your upper outer arm, just below your shoulder joint. No other joints are affected. You have not noticed any swelling, heat or redness of your right shoulder. You have not had any neck pain. There is no tingling or numbness in your right arm or hand. You have been well in yourself otherwise and have not been feverish. You are right-handed, so the shoulder problem has been even more difficult to manage. You now brush your teeth and eat using your left hand. You have found it increasingly hard to work as your right shoulder has been so painful. You have been using your left arm to steer and try not to use your right arm, changing gears by taking your left hand off the steering wheel momentarily. Even getting dressed in the morning has become difficult, particularly if there are any front fastenings. You are not going to the toilet more frequently and you are not excessively thirsty.

Ideas, concerns and expectations – You think you may have strained your shoulder but you are not sure how you did this. You think it is best to rest your shoulder. You have heard from a friend that acupuncture can help shoulder pain and want to ask the doctor about this. A couple of your customers have commented on your taking your hand off the steering wheel to change gears and you are worried that you may be reported. You know that you should probably stop driving at the moment but you need the income. You are hoping that the doctor will arrange an X-ray and may be able to offer you some treatment – some acupuncture or an injection.

First words spoken to doctor – *"Sorry to bother you, doctor, but my right shoulder has been giving me so much trouble, I can't sleep and driving my taxi* *is getting to be a real problem. I know that I shouldn't be taking the Brufen but it's the only thing that helps the pain. It's really starting to get me down."*

Past medical history – You had an ulcer just beyond your stomach in your small bowel when you were 33 years old which required surgery. You have not had any further problems with ulcers since then. You are otherwise fit and well.

Drug history – You have been taking ibuprofen, which you bought at the supermarket, for the last 4 weeks. To start with you only took one or two 200 mg tablets a day. But as the shoulder pain worsened you started to take more, and are now taking two 200 mg tablets four times a day (which you know is more than the maximum it says on the packet). You did try paracetamol at first, but this did not seem to give much relief.

Social history – You work as a self-employed taxi driver. You have not smoked since you were a teenager. You used to drink heavily but after your ulcer surgery you stopped completely. You live with your wife and grown up son.

Family history – There is no family history of diabetes or joint problems in your immediate family.

- Having read the information given to the simulated patient, what do you now think this station is testing?
- Make notes or discuss your thoughts with a colleague before you turn the page.

Review your approach to this station:

Tested at this station:

1. Generic communication skills
2. History taking skills
3. Physical examination skills
4. Reaching a shared management plan

Domain 1 – Interpersonal skills

Generic communication skills

In the marking scheme for the CSA, each of the three domains – interpersonal skills; data gathering, examination and clinical assessment skills; clinical management skills – carry equal weight. At this station there is no specific communication issue (e.g. such as the patient being angry, talkative or with a hearing impairment). Indeed, the primary nature of this case is testing physical examination skills. However, you must still be able to demonstrate effective communication skills during the consultation to score marks, and so the list below is a recap on some of these generic skills:

- Remember the importance of non-verbal communication, including body language and eye contact.
- Always start with open questions before moving on to more specific closed questions.
- Use paraphrasing, checking and summarizing to show that you are actively listening.
- Pick up on, and respond to, cues that the patient gives – such as his awareness that he should not be driving in his current condition.
- Always remember to ask about the patient's ideas, concerns and expectations. Does he have any thoughts about what is going on with his shoulder? Are there any particular concerns? What is he hoping will happen from coming to see you today?
- When giving information, such as explaining a diagnosis, avoid talking at length. Instead 'chunk and check' – i.e. give information in manageable chunks, then check the patient's understanding before you move on.
- Avoid medical jargon and use lay terminology – appropriate to the patient – when explaining diagnosis and treatment options.
- Try to stay patient-centred during the consultation – in other words identify the patient's agenda and address it.
- Give patients the opportunity to raise any other issues which they might not at first have mentioned – *"Is there anything else I can help you with today?"*
- Encourage patients to ask questions at the end of the consultation – *"Is there anything you would like to ask?"*
- Check understanding of the management plan, including follow-up – Can he say what the plan is that you have jointly agreed?

Domain 2 – Data gathering, examination and clinical assessment skills

History taking skills

When a patient presents with a painful joint you need to feel confident that you have excluded conditions requiring immediate action (e.g. septic arthritis or dislocation). You should also rule out other red flags that might prompt referral to a specialist. Next, you need to identify the likely structural origin of the pain (e.g. in this case, neck, shoulder or elsewhere). Finally, if you feel that the problem is indeed originating from the shoulder, you should try and differentiate between the common shoulder injuries (see Knowledge-base). A focused history, together with examination, will help you do all this:

- He says that his right shoulder has been giving him trouble – can he say more about this?
- Where precisely is the pain: neck, shoulder or arm? Can he show you?
- Any history of trauma? Does the patient do any heavy exercise involving his arms?
- Is he well in himself otherwise – any fevers or general malaise?
- Any weight loss or problems with his breathing? Does he have pain at rest? Is there any history of cancer?
- Has his shoulder ever been dislocated? Does it feel unstable as though it might become dislocated?
- Has his shoulder swollen up? Has the skin over the joint been red or hot?
- Are any other joints affected?
- Has he had problems with his joints in the past?
- Is the pain worse first thing in the morning or later on in the day, or is there no pattern?
- Do any of the patient's immediate family suffer from joint problems (such as rheumatoid arthritis)?
- Any eye problems or pain passing urine? (Reiter's syndrome)
- Is the patient left or right-handed?
- What effect has the shoulder problem had on his day-to-day life? He says that driving his taxi has become a real problem – can he say more about how it is affecting his work?
- During the history you should also try and exclude referred angina or diaphragmatic irritation as causes of his shoulder pain.
- This patient has a history of peptic ulcer disease and he has been taking regular NSAIDs. You need to make sure that he has not experienced any symptoms suggesting recurrence of an ulcer or gastrointestinal bleed:
  - Any heartburn or indigestion recently?
  - Any abdominal pain?
  - Does he feel nauseous or has he vomited?
  - Has he seen any blood in his stools or have his stools changed colour such that they are now dark and tarry?

Physical examination skills

The GP curriculum lists examination of the shoulder as one of the psycho-motor skills that you should be able competently to demonstrate. Indeed, physical examination is the 'nub' of this case. With any joint examination a rough guide is: look, feel, move (active, passive and against resistance):

- Always explain the nature of the examination to the patient and gain consent.
- You can often pick up clues even before the start of the formal examination. This patient enters the room with his right arm immobile, flexed at the elbow and held against his body, which gives you an idea about his loss of function.
- Ask the patient to take his top off so you can examine the shoulder adequately.
- Inspection – both from in front and behind, look for signs of deformity, swelling, asymmetry, redness and muscle wasting.
- Palpation – palpate the sternoclavicular, acromioclavicular and glenohumeral joints, looking for signs of localized tenderness (see Knowledgebase). The tendon of biceps is palpated anteriorly in the bicipital groove between the humeral greater and lesser tubercles.
- Assessing movement – as a quick screening test ask the patient to put his hands behind his head and then to place them in the small of his back. This is a gross test of a variety of movements at the shoulder joint, including flexion, extension, internal and external rotation.
- Assessing movement – active movement. In turn, ask the patient to flex, extend, abduct, adduct, externally and internally rotate the shoulder as far as he can. For abduction, you can fix the scapula to isolate glenohumeral joint function.
- Assessing movement – passive movement. If there are limitations of active movement, then see whether you can passively move the joint beyond the limitations found on active movement. Frozen shoulder problems usually do not allow any further passive movement whereas rotator cuff injuries often do.
- Assessing movement – painful arc. Pain on abduction between 70° and 120° suggests rotator cuff injury, as does pain on abduction that is worse against resistance.
- Assess for crepitus during the examination.

There are no abnormalities on inspection apart from how the patient holds his right arm on entering the room. See Information given to simulated patient for further positive findings.

Domain 3 – Clinical management skills

Reaching a shared management plan (overlap with domain 1)

This patient's history and examination findings suggest a glenohumeral joint disorder, namely frozen shoulder (adhesive capsulitis). However, mixed shoulder problems are common and the exact diagnostic category often does not change what is primarily conservative management in a general practice setting, namely: analgesia, physiotherapy and encouragement to return to normal activities as early as possible:

- Explain the probable diagnosis – how the capsule around the shoulder joint can become swollen and thickened and lead to pain and restricted movement.
- Given advice on prognosis – prepare the patient for a potentially protracted course, as symptoms can last for 2 or 3 years.
- Encourage self-management of his condition. Explain that keeping the shoulder mobile is a key goal. Gentle shoulder exercises several times a day will help. The exercises will involve some discomfort but are important to prevent muscle wasting.
- Pain management is a key element to facilitate mobilization and allow him to sleep better. You need to explain the risks of internal bleeding with NSAIDs and negotiate their use. Has he thought about trying regular maximum strength paracetamol, with a topical NSAID gel? He could then reserve oral ibuprofen for occasional use if the pain is particularly bad. You could also consider giving him a proton pump inhibitor (PPI) – e.g. omeprazole 20 mg OD – for gastroprotection to cover his use of oral NSAIDs. Explain how he would need to discontinue NSAIDs if he started to suffer from indigestion.
- Offer the patient other treatment options including steroid injections and physiotherapy. Physiotherapy will involve exercises and possibly heat treatment. Explain that the evidence for both treatments' long term effectiveness is weak, but they may help with short term relief. What does he think about these options?
- Explain that X-rays and blood tests are not indicated unless there are worrying (red flag) signs, and reassure him that he has none.
- Encourage early return to normal activities, if possible.
- However, at present it appears that his restricted movement renders him unsafe to drive. You should be explicit in your advice that he has a legal duty to inform the DVLA and must refrain from driving at present. (See GMC guidelines in Further reading). This advice has major implications for the patient and you need to explore his response sensitively and empathetically.
- He is reluctant to stop working due to financial pressures. You could offer to give him a sick note (Med 3) as he may be entitled to incapacity benefit at the lower rate once he is off work through illness for 4 days or more. The current rate is £57.65 per week (see Further reading).
- The patient wants to know about acupuncture treatment for his shoulder. You can advise him that there is little evidence either to confirm or refute the effectiveness of acupuncture for shoulder problems, but that it may improve pain and function for a few weeks.
- Frozen shoulder is five times more common in people with diabetes mellitus, but he has no symptoms and no family history, so this possibility is unlikely to need further investigation.

Knowledge-base – Diagnosis of shoulder problems

Adapted with permission from Oxford Shoulder and Elbow Clinic shoulder diagnosis flowchart. www.oxfordshoulderandelbowclinic.org.uk.

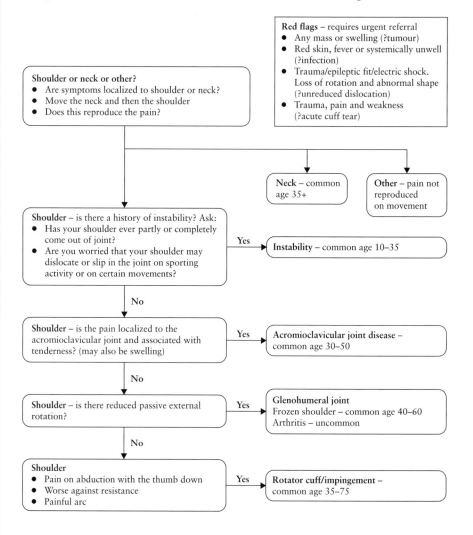

Red flags – requires urgent referral
- Any mass or swelling (?tumour)
- Red skin, fever or systemically unwell (?infection)
- Trauma/epileptic fit/electric shock. Loss of rotation and abnormal shape (?unreduced dislocation)
- Trauma, pain and weakness (?acute cuff tear)

Shoulder or neck or other?
- Are symptoms localized to shoulder or neck?
- Move the neck and then the shoulder
- Does this reproduce the pain?

Neck – common age 35+

Other – pain not reproduced on movement

Shoulder – is there a history of instability? Ask:
- Has your shoulder ever partly or completely come out of joint?
- Are you worried that your shoulder may dislocate or slip in the joint on sporting activity or on certain movements?

Yes → Instability – common age 10–35

No

Shoulder – is the pain localized to the acromioclavicular joint and associated with tenderness? (may also be swelling)

Yes → Acromioclavicular joint disease – common age 30–50

No

Shoulder – is there reduced passive external rotation?

Yes → Glenohumeral joint
Frozen shoulder – common age 40–60
Arthritis – uncommon

No

Shoulder
- Pain on abduction with the thumb down
- Worse against resistance
- Painful arc

Yes → Rotator cuff/impingement – common age 35–75

- Referral to a specialist is indicated if:
  - Red flags are present (see above).
  - There is a history of joint instability.
  - There is significant disability and no improvement in pain over a 6-month period, despite conservative management.
  - There is diagnostic uncertainty.
  - Surgery may be considered if conservative treatment is unsuccessful.

Take home messages

- Shoulder problems are common, can be protracted, and mainly involve conservative management in primary care.
- Always exclude red flags when patients present with joint pain.
- Remember that at each CSA station you need to score marks in all three domains.

Ideas for further revision

Examination of a joint lends itself to inclusion in the CSA. Be sure that you have a good framework for examining the shoulder, knee, hip and back, and can apply the principles to any joint examination.

Further reading

GMC guidance – Confidentiality: Protecting and Providing Information. Frequently Asked Questions: Patients driving/DVLA, question 17. April 2004. www.gmc-uk.org/guidance/current/library/confidentiality_faq.asp#q17.

Information on Incapacity Benefit (for those not eligible for Statutory Sick Pay – e.g. the self-employed). www.jobcentreplus.gov.uk.

Maguire P. *Communication Skills for Doctors*. London: Arnold, 2000.

Mitchell C, Adebajo A, Hay E, Carr A. Shoulder pain: diagnosis and management in primary care. *BMJ* 2005;**331**:1124–1128. www.bmj.com.

Munro JF, Campbell IW (eds). *Macleod's Clinical Examination*, 10th edn. Churchill Livingstone, Edinburgh, 2000.

NHS National Library for Health Clinical Knowledge Summaries – frozen shoulder. www.cks.library.nhs.uk/clinical_knowledge.

Oxford Shoulder and Elbow Clinic. www.oxfordshoulderandelbowclinic.org.uk.

Information given to candidates

Fatima Ahmed is an Urdu speaker who rarely comes to the surgery. At previous appointments for minor illnesses family members have acted as interpreters.

She is 38 years old and married with three children.

She attended hospital 8 weeks ago to have a vulval cyst removed. The discharge letter from the gynaecology team states:

Dear GP,

Mrs Ahmed attended for a planned procedure under general anaesthetic to remove a vulval cyst. This went well and the histology shows no worrying findings. However, during the procedure there appeared to be a fistula in the posterior vaginal wall communicating with the rectum, which was discharging a small amount of pus into the vagina. The surgeons kindly reviewed the patient later on the ward. They felt that there may indeed be a small fistula but that it would probably close on its own. They discussed options with the patient and it was agreed to 'wait and see'. If things are no better in 4–6 weeks' time then please refer her back to the surgeons for further management.

When the patient enters the room she has a trained interpreter with her – Mrs Lone – who was booked by one of the receptionists.

- What do you think this station is testing?
- Make notes or discuss your thoughts with a colleague before you read on.

Plan your approach to this station:

Information given to simulated patient

Basic details – You are Fatima Ahmed, an Urdu speaker and 38-year-old mother of three, originally from Pakistan. You came to the UK when you were 34 years old to join your husband, who had moved here the year before. You are not able to speak much English at all, but you do understand simple spoken English quite well.

Appearance and behaviour – You are wearing a headscarf. You are softly spoken and do not make much eye contact. You answer the doctor's questions in a direct manner – through the interpreter – although at times you appear to be embarrassed at discussing these personal matters.

History
Freely divulged to doctor – You went to hospital about 2 months ago to have a cyst removed. Soon after leaving hospital you noticed a small amount of yellow discharge from your vagina which has occurred on and off since then. It has still not cleared up so you decided to visit the GP. Your husband is away on family business in Pakistan at the moment, so you came down to the surgery on your own.

Divulged to doctor if specifically asked – The doctors at the hospital told you that the procedure went well and that they would send the results to your GP, after looking at the cyst under a microscope. You also had to see some different doctors back on the ward because there was a 'channel' which should not have been there. You did not really understand what they meant or where the 'channel' was. You have not been feverish or felt unwell. You have never had any sexually transmitted infections. You had a healthy sex life with your husband before you attended the hospital but have not had intercourse since, due to the operation and the subsequent vaginal discharge. Apart from your husband, you have not had any other sexual partners since you were married 12 years ago. You have not had any pelvic or abdominal pain, or any pain on intercourse. Your periods are regular – the last one was 2 weeks ago. You have been opening your bowels and passing urine without any problems. You have not felt down or depressed recently.

Ideas, concerns and expectations – You had noticed the cyst several months ago and had been glad to have the operation to get rid of it. When you were in hospital it was difficult to fully understand the doctors as they used long words. But one of the nurses spoke Urdu and would come and see you to explain what the doctors had said. But this nurse was not around when the different doctors came to talk about the 'channel'. You are worried that the discharge has not cleared up. You are hoping the doctor today will explain what the 'channel' is and where the discharge is coming from, and refer you back to the hospital.

First words spoken to doctor – "I have come to the doctor's as I still have a discharge."

Past medical history – You attended hospital in Pakistan for your first child's birth, but since then have not been back in a hospital until the removal of the cyst on your vulva (the external parts of the female genitals) 2 months ago. All three births have been uncomplicated vaginal deliveries. You are otherwise fit and well.

Drug history – You had 2 week's supply of antibiotics after you left hospital a month ago. You do not take any regular medication. As far as you know you are not allergic to any medication.

Social history – You live with your husband and three children – all girls under 10. You were fairly well educated in Pakistan, although your spoken English has always been poor. You work as a counsellor at the local Pakistani community support centre 3 days a week. Your extended family lives nearby and offers a great deal of support, including childcare. You have a good circle of friends who are all from the local Urdu-speaking community. Your husband has his own wholesale business which he runs with two of his cousins. You do not drink alcohol or smoke.

Family history – There are no major illnesses in your immediate family.

Information given to simulated interpreter

Basic details – You are Mrs Lone, a 55-year-old professional interpreter who speaks Urdu. You work for the local primary care trust but live in another city, 40 miles away. You have just met the patient for the first time in the waiting room.

Appearance and behaviour – You are professionally dressed and solely interpret the doctor's questions and the patient's responses.

- Having read the information given to the simulated patient and interpreter, what do you now think this station is testing?
- Make notes or discuss your thoughts with a colleague before you turn the page.

Review your approach to this station:

Tested at this station:

1. Conducting a consultation using an interpreter
2. History taking skills
3. Negotiating a shared management plan

Domain 1 – Interpersonal skills

Conducting a consultation using an interpreter

Ideally an interpreter should be as unobtrusive as possible. However, the consultation dynamic will undoubtedly change significantly. You need to try and minimize this effect as much as possible:

- Set up the seating arrangement in a triangle, with both yourself and the patient able to see the interpreter.
- Introduce yourself and the interpreter to the patient.
- Explain what the role of the interpreter will be during the consultation and reassure the patient that what is discussed is confidential – for both yourself and the interpreter.
- At the start, tell the interpreter to ask for clarification from you, if she does not fully understand what you are asking her to translate.
- Speak directly to the patient, observe her reactions, and maintain eye contact to allow you to respond with non-verbal recognition to the interpreter's translation (e.g. head nods, smiles).
- Use the second person when conducting the interview – i.e. 'What do *you* think about *your* problem?' rather than 'What does *she* think about *her* problem?' This encourages you to have the conversation with the patient, rather than with the interpreter.
- Use unambiguous words and avoid medical jargon.
- Be alert to whether the interpreter appears to be answering for the patient, rather than translating what is said. This is less likely with a trained interpreter.
- Be aware that if the interpreter is from the same local community as the patient, then it may be difficult for the patient to speak openly.

Domain 2 – Data gathering, examination and clinical assessment skills

History taking skills

You need to use the skills outlined above while taking a comprehensive history of the patient's complaint:

- Open questions and exploration of the patient's ideas, concerns and expectations should help you understand her perspective on events.
- Acknowledge that it can be difficult talking about these matters, but that it is important to try and understand about the discharge.
- More specific closed questions will allow you to obtain a comprehensive history of her current symptoms:
  - What is the discharge like? Does she have to wear pads?

○ Is the discharge there all the time or does it come and go?
○ Any fever or weight loss, or lack of appetite?
○ Any pain in her tummy, or lower down at the front?
○ Any back pain?
○ Any pain during sexual intercourse?
○ When was her last period – any different from usual? Any inter-menstrual or post-coital bleeding?
○ Any problems when she opens her bowels? Or urinates?
○ Has she ever had any sexually transmitted infections?
○ Has she ever suffered from any other medical problems? Any previous operations? Any problems with previous deliveries?
○ Any family history of bowel problems?
● Vaginal discharge should usually prompt you to take a full sexual history (see Examination 1 Station 5). However, in this case, as you already know about the fistula, you may feel this is not necessary.

Physical examination

Time is particularly short at this station since all dialogue needs to be translated by the interpreter. The examiner will intervene if you start to mention physical examination and tell you to assume that you have conducted a full abdominal and pelvic examination, including swabs, and that the findings are normal apart from a small amount of yellow discharge seen in the vagina.

Domain 3 – Clinical management skills

Negotiating a shared management plan

The key management action point for this station is to offer to refer the patient back to the surgeons for further investigation of her fistula. However, you also need to explain to the patient about the fistula findings:

● The patient is embarrassed at the personal nature of the discussion. You should be alert to this and recognize that her embarrassment may be increased by cultural or social influences.
● She has asked about the histology results for the removed cyst. You can reassure her that these are fine.
● Explaining the fistula findings may be more easily done by drawing a simple diagram.
● You should be honest and explain that you are not sure why the fistula is there, but that – if she would like you to – you could ask the surgeons to see her again to investigate this further.
● When explaining the problem and management options, ask her to repeat back what has been said, to check understanding.
● Repeatedly encourage the patient to ask questions.
● Would it be useful if someone came with her to her next appointment, to offer support?
● And if possible, could the interpreter liaise with the patient to ensure that the same interpreter is present at any future appointment with the surgeons?

Knowledge-base – Interviewing with an interpreter

Key points

- Address the patient in the second person.
- Talk directly to the patient.
- Keep control of the consultation.
- Pause frequently.
- Appear attentive when patient responds.
- Respond to non-verbal cues.
- Check patient's understanding.
- Make use of written material.

From Phelan & Parkman (1995). Reproduced with permission from BMJ Publishing Group.

Further points

- If you know that an interpreter will be present, try and book a longer appointment.
- Be aware that some hospital and primary care trusts have contracts with language lines, where interpreters are available 24 h a day, via the telephone, in most languages.
- At the end of the consultation you could ask the interpreter for feedback on the communication issues – could you have made the interpreter's job easier?

Take home messages

- When conducting consultations using an interpreter, try and build rapport using the physical set-up of the room, good eye contact and non-verbal responses.
- Allow patients using interpreters repeated opportunities to ask questions and seek clarification.
- Drawing explanatory diagrams is often useful.

Ideas for further revision

The GP curriculum states that one of the learning objectives for trainees is to develop communication skills, including working with interpreters to deal with patients from diverse backgrounds. If you work in an ethnically diverse area, then you should have ample opportunity to practise these skills. If not, then you could ask your programme director to arrange teaching sessions with simulated patients and interpreters. You could also contact trained interpreters who work in healthcare settings, to try to understand the various issues that arise within these consultations.

Further reading

Adams K. Making the best use of health advocates and interpreters. *BMJ Career Focus* 2002;**325**:S9a. http://careerfocus.bmj.com.

Phelan M, Parkman S. How to do it: Work with an interpreter. *BMJ* 1995;**311**:555–557. www.bmj.com.

RCGP curriculum statement 10.1 – Women's health and RCGP curriculum statement 3.4 – Promoting equality and valuing diversity. www.rcgp.org.uk.

Information given to candidates

Tony Barrett is a 58-year-old patient who rarely visits the surgery.

He was seen 7 days ago by your colleague with a subconjunctival haemorrhage in his left eye. There was no pain or any visual problems reported by the patient at that time.

Full examination of his eyes, including acuity, fundoscopy, eye movements and pupillary response were all normal. His BP was 128/82.

His records state that he had asked if he needed to take time off work for his subconjunctival haemorrhage, and that your colleague advised him that this was not necessary.

You note that he was seen on two occasions 4 months ago with a bad back, which gradually resolved with symptomatic relief and physiotherapy. He received Med 3 sick notes for a total of 6 weeks during that episode.

As the patient enters the consultation room he says, "All I need is a sick note for my eye for last week, but I don't understand why I've been waiting 40 bloody minutes."

If you decide to examine the patient today, assume that BP is normal and there is no abnormality of either eye.

- What do you think this station is testing?
- Make notes or discuss your thoughts with a colleague before you read on.

Plan your approach to this station:

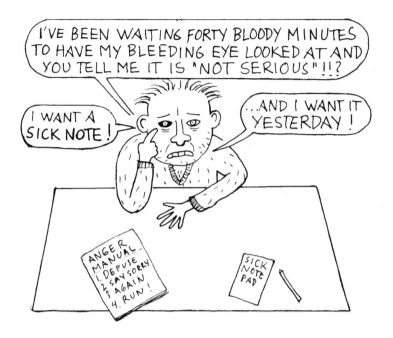

Information given to simulated patient

Basic details – You are Tony Barrett a Caucasian 58-year-old single man who works as a fork-lift truck driver.

Appearance and behaviour – You are angry at having to wait 40 min to see the doctor today. However, if the doctor is understanding and apologetic you will soon calm down and even apologize yourself for being 'a bit rude' when you came in.

History

Freely divulged to doctor – You woke up last week with what looked like blood in your left eye. Nothing like that had ever happened to you before so you booked an emergency appointment to see the doctor. She checked you over and told you it was 'a bleed into the eye'. You were due to work two night shifts starting that night, but when you got home you thought it would be best to take it easy and you called in sick. You went back to work after missing those two night shifts as the eye seemed to be improving. Now your work wants a doctor's sick note to cover the time you were off.

Divulged to doctor if specifically asked – You have not had any pain or problems with your vision in either eye. You remember the other doctor saying that you did not need to take any time off work, but after you had walked home you thought that 'to be on the safe side' you should stay at home. The red patch of blood in your left eye gradually disappeared over the following week. You have never had anything go into your eyes and your work is not an environment where this happens. You have not suffered from any headaches.

Ideas, concerns and expectations – Although you felt that the doctor checked you over thoroughly last week, you were worried when she said that you had 'a bleed into the eye' and did not quite understand the diagnosis. Four months ago you took 6 weeks off work with a bad back, and had to see the sickness manager about this. You felt under pressure to return to work then, and you were told that he would be keeping an eye on your sick leave. You are afraid that work may target you for redundancy because of your time off and you think having a doctor's certificate will help matters. You believe that you are entitled to a sick note, even if you have only taken two night shifts off, as you think things looked pretty bad in your eye last week. Initially, you will not be happy if the doctor says that they cannot give you a standard sick note, but if the doctor acknowledges your worries about work and clearly explains the situation regarding issuing a retrospective sick note, you will accept this. As a compromise, you would be prepared to pay for a private sick note if the doctor offers this as an option.

First words spoken to doctor – "All I need is a sick note for my eye for last week, but I don't understand why I've been waiting 40 bloody minutes."

Past medical history – You strained your back 4 months ago and were off work for 6 weeks. You took painkillers and saw a physiotherapist privately, which helped considerably, and you have not had any problems since going back to work. You are otherwise fit and well.

Drug history – You do not take any regular medication and have no drug allergies.

Social history – You live on your own. You have never been married but have a close group of friends from work and the local brass band, which you have been a member of since you were 12 years old. You do shift work in an engineering plant, mostly using a fork-lift truck to stack the metal sheet products that your company produces. You stopped smoking when you were 24 years old and drink one or two pints of beer on Friday and Saturday nights.

Family history – There are no major health problems in your family. As far as you know, no-one in your family has had glaucoma or any eye problems other than wearing glasses for reading.

- Having read the information given to the simulated patient, what do you now think this station is testing?
- Make notes or discuss your thoughts with a colleague before you turn the page.

Review your approach to this station:

Tested at this station:

1. Dealing with an angry patient
2. History taking skills
3. Dealing with a sick note request

Domain 1 – Interpersonal skills

Dealing with an angry patient

Dealing with patients' emotions is a key skill which can be readily tested in the CSA:

- This patient is angry at being kept waiting 40 min. As a first step, acknowledge his anger and make a sincere apology for the delay.
- Avoid the temptation to blame someone or something else for the delay – e.g. *"I'm sorry but the receptionist keeps making mistakes with our new booking system."*
- Apologizing – repeatedly if necessary – demonstrates that you are prepared to take responsibility for the delay, rather than sidestepping or dismissing it.
- If he continues to be angry, then ask whether there is anything else upsetting him today.
- Be aware of your own emotional response to such situations. You may feel under attack and angry with the patient for taking their frustrations out on you. You need to have strategies for dealing with these emotions to allow you to remain professional and patient-centred during the consultation.
- Avoid responses to angry patients that can lead to further confrontation or an escalation of the situation – e.g. being defensive or contradictory – *"Well the computer shows that you have actually only been waiting 33 minutes."*
- You will have some difficult negotiating to do regarding the sick note request later on in the consultation, so it is all the more important to fully address, and defuse, the patient's anger at the start.
- If at any time you feel threatened or physically intimidated by an angry patient, you should end the consultation and remove yourself from the room.

Domain 2 – Data gathering, examination and clinical assessment skills

History taking skills

Once the patient has calmed down, you need to take a history to see if there have been any developments since your colleague saw him last week. You also need to explore his understanding and any concerns he may have about his eye:

- He wants a sick note to cover him for last week. For your benefit, could he recap why he came to see the doctor then?
- What is his understanding of the problem with his eye last week?

- Since then has he experienced any new symptoms, including:
  - Headaches
  - Visual problems (e.g. double vision, blurred vision)
  - Eye pain
  - Soreness or irritation
  - A sensation that there is something in his eye.
- Is there any history of anything going into his eye, e.g. at work?
- How have things progressed with the blood he saw in the white of his left eye last week?
- This patient was worried last week when he heard that he had 'a bleed into the eye'. Was there anything he was particularly worried about? Does he understand that although it may have looked dramatic, the condition is not serious?

Physical examination

His records state that when your colleague examined the patient last week there was nothing to find except a subconjunctival haemorrhage in his left eye. You are told that today there is no abnormality of either eye and that his BP is normal.

Domain 3 – Clinical management skills

Dealing with a sick note request

The patient wants a sick note for last week, even though your colleague advised him that he did not need to take any time off work. Trying to understand why he wants a sick note will help you address his concerns and help you to negotiate an outcome that is acceptable to both of you:

- Why does he feel he needs a sick note for last week?
- Has his employer asked him to obtain one?
- Is he concerned that having time off without a sick note will affect how he is treated at work?
- Has he had much time off work recently through illness?
- Did he discuss obtaining a sick note when he saw the doctor last week?
- You can advise him that employers should not routinely ask for a doctor's sick note for the first 7 days of an illness, as employees are able to self-certify for this period.
- You should explain that since it was not you who saw the patient last week, you are only able to issue a sick note retrospectively on a standard Med 5 form if the report from the doctor who did see the patient supports the advice to refrain from work (see Knowledge-base). But, as the patient remembers, the advice last week was that he did not need to take time off.
- However, the patient appears not to have fully understood the diagnosis last week and was concerned about 'a bleed into the eye', so one option would be to offer to write a private sick note. Does he realize that this will incur a fee? What does he think about this as a way forward?
- You may be reluctant to issue any type of sick note if you think this would undermine your colleague. However, there has clearly been some misunderstanding in that the patient genuinely felt that his problem was significant.

- In this scenario there is no one right answer on how to deal with the request for a sick note, but a good candidate would fully explore the patient's concerns, make sure that he understood the nature of the diagnosis, and empathetically explain the situation and options regarding the issuing of sick notes in this case.

Knowledge-base – Issuing sick notes

Reference – Department for Work and Pensions guidance.

More commonly used	Med 3 – statement of incapacity for work	<ul><li>You must have examined the patient on the day, or the day before, issuing a Med 3</li><li>Closed certificates – those for which you complete the 'until' section and give a specific date for return to work. May be up to 14 days from issue date</li><li>Open certificates – those for which you complete the 'for' section (e.g. 'for 2 weeks'), with no specific date given for return to work. The implication is that you plan to review the patient</li><li>For the first 6 months, you can issue a Med 3 for a period of up to 6 months from your examination. Thereafter, there is no limit on how long you can issue it for; indeed, you can put 'until further notice', if appropriate</li></ul>
	Med 5 – special statement of incapacity for work	<ul><li>This allows you to supply evidence of incapacity for work for an earlier period, either based on a previous examination by you, or from a report by another doctor</li><li>You can use a report from another doctor to support an opinion that your patient is incapable of work only if:<ul><li>○ The report was issued in the last month</li><li>○ The certificate you issue does not cover a forward period of > 1 month</li></ul></li></ul>
Less commonly used	Med 4 – statement used for patients undergoing the Personal Capability Assessment	<ul><li>The patient will have received a letter from the Department for Work and Pensions (DWP) advising them that the Personal Capability Assessment is to be applied. This is usually after 28 weeks of incapacity. The letter asks patients to obtain a Med 4 from their doctor</li><li>You are required to detail:<ul><li>○ Diagnosis of the main incapacitating condition</li><li>○ Other relevant medical conditions</li><li>○ Disabling effects of the condition</li><li>○ Current treatment and progress</li><li>○ Advice you have given the patient regarding their ability to perform their usual occupation</li></ul></li></ul>
	Med 6 – statement offering further information on diagnosis	<ul><li>If you have not entered a diagnosis on form Med 3, 4 or 5 as precisely as the rules require, you should notify the local DWP office by also sending a Med 6 form to them</li><li>Useful if you think that it could be prejudicial to the patient's well-being if you issue a certificate to them with the true diagnosis</li></ul>

Less commonly used	DS 1500 – 'special rules' speeds up application for Disability Living Allowance (DLA) and other benefits	• You can issue a DS 1500 if you think the patient may be suffering from a potentially terminal illness • Terminal illness is defined as a progressive disease where death can reasonably be expected within 6 months

For Med 3, 4 and 5 certificates:

- Ensure that you record an accurate diagnosis – terms which do not relate to a specific disease or disablement, such as 'bereavement' or 'pregnancy', should not be used.
- Any replacement certificate (e.g. if the original is lost or stolen) must be marked 'duplicate' and should be provided by the doctor who issued the original certificate.
- These certificates are for Social Security purposes only and should not be used for anything other than Statutory Sick Pay or Social Security benefit purposes.

Take home messages

- You need to feel confident managing an angry patient both in everyday practice and in an exam setting such as the CSA.
- Acknowledging the patient's anger and apologizing can help diffuse the situation and allow you to move on to address their presenting complaint.
- Doctors need to work within the statutory framework governing the issuing of sick notes.

Ideas for further revision

In the CSA you might have to deal with patients displaying a range of challenging emotions or behaviours. Think about, and practise with colleagues, how you would approach patients presenting with: distress, anger, a dismissive attitude, reticence or over familiarity.

Further reading

Department for Work and Pensions. Medical evidence for Statutory Sick Pay, Statutory Maternity pay and Social Security Incapacity Benefit purposes: A guide for registered medical practitioners. Revised August 2004. www.dwp.gov.uk/medical/guides_detailed.asp.

Maguire P. *Communication Skills for Doctors*. London: Arnold, 2000.

Examination 2: Station 10

Warning – *readers may find some of the language used in this station offensive.*

Information given to candidates

> Jim Nelson is a 38-year-old obese patient who suffers from hypertension.
>
> He has been taking amlodipine 5 mg OD for the last 6 months. When he saw the nurse for a blood pressure check 2 weeks ago it was 138/80. His BMI was found to be 34.
>
> His records state that he is a smoker.

The first thing the patient says when he enters the room is, "Doctor, I need something stronger for my indigestion. I had a large Chinky meal last week and that set it off, and the other day after eating a samosa from the Paki shop things were really bad."

- What do you think this station is testing?
- Make notes or discuss your thoughts with a colleague before you read on.

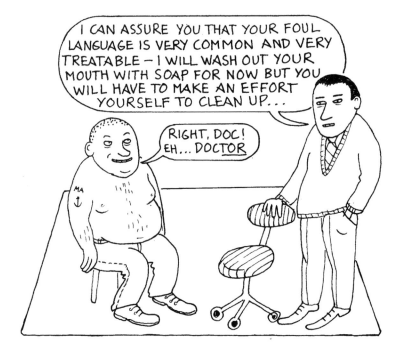

Plan your approach to this station:

Information given to simulated patient

Basic details – You are Jim Nelson, a Caucasian 38-year-old single man, originally from Glasgow.

Appearance and behaviour – You are overweight. If the doctor challenges you about the language you use in your opening statement then initially you will be surprised – you did not think that such words would cause offence. So long as the doctor is polite and does not go on at length about what you have said, you will apologize and say that you will try not to use such words again. Overall, you will not be too bothered by the doctor's comments about your language – you really just want to get your indigestion sorted out.

History
Freely divulged to doctor – You have had intermittent heartburn for about 5 years now. Things have been worse in the last 3 or 4 months. Last year you only had problems two or three times a month, whereas now you are getting symptoms three or four times a week. You feel an uncomfortable sensation in your upper abdomen and behind your breastbone, usually after meals. Lying down makes things worse. You have never been to the doctor's before about your indigestion. You are otherwise well.

Divulged to doctor if specifically asked – In the past, your symptoms settled with antacids such as Rennies; however, recently they do not seem to help as much. Things are worse after large meals and at night. You have not felt nauseous or vomited. You have no problems swallowing. You have never seen any blood when you open your bowels. Your stools have not been darker or black. Your appetite is fine and you have not lost any weight. Your pain never radiates into your arms and you do not experience any pain when you exert yourself, such as climbing a flight of stairs. You do not suffer from shortness of breath. You have not had any time off work due to your symptoms. You do not feel particularly stressed at the moment.

Ideas, concerns and expectations – When you first speak to the doctor you do not mean to upset or insult anyone by your choice of words, but are just trying to describe where and when the indigestion was particularly bad. Where you grew up in Glasgow everyone used these terms without people commenting. You are not concerned that your indigestion is anything serious, but it is worse now and the symptoms are really unpleasant. You know that you should probably cut out spicy foods. You are hoping the doctor can prescribe something to help.

First words spoken to doctor – "Doctor, I need something stronger for my indigestion. I had a large Chinky meal last week and that set it off, and the other day after eating a samosa from the Paki shop things were really bad."

Past medical history – You were told that you had high blood pressure 6 months ago, after it was checked by the doctor and nurse several times. But the tablets seem to be working and the nurse was happy with your blood pressure when you had it checked a couple of weeks ago.

Drug history – You have been taking one tablet in the morning for your blood pressure – amlodipine 5 mg – for the last 6 months. You have been taking antacids, such as Rennies, which you buy at the chemist, for about 5 years, although you are using them more frequently now. You are not allergic to any medication.

Social history – You work shifts in the local meat packing factory. You smoke 20 cigarettes a day and drink a couple of pints most nights when you are not working. Your brother is a member of the British National Party (BNP – a right-wing political party advocating resettlement of immigrants living in Britain back to their 'lands of ethnic origin'). You are not a BNP member but you are sympathetic to some of its views on immigration. You live with your brother in an almost exclusively white council estate.

Family history – There is no history of serious medical problems in your immediate family.

- Having read the information given to the simulated patient, what do you now think this station is testing?
- Make notes or discuss your thoughts with a colleague before you turn the page.

Review your approach to this station:

Tested at this station:

1. Understanding of equality and diversity issues: challenging a patient's racist language
2. History taking skills
3. Reaching a shared management plan

Domain 1 – Interpersonal skills

Understanding of equality and diversity issues: challenging a patient's racist language

This is a particularly sensitive and difficult station. The patient has used words that are derogatory and offensive. 'Chinky' is considered an ethnic slur for Chinese people and 'Paki' has pejorative connotations and is used as a term of abuse towards those from the Indian sub-continent. As such this language, even when describing food or shops rather than people, is indirect racist comment and therefore unacceptable:

- It would be easy to ignore the patient's terminology and focus on his physical complaint. However, doing so would be an abdication of your responsibility to promote equality and diversity and to challenge discriminatory language.
- The GP curriculum states that issues of equality and diversity are at the heart of the work of GPs and that you should recognize, respect, value and harness difference. Indeed, the curriculum learning outcomes state that a GP should be able to challenge behaviour that infringes the rights of others and recognize and take action to address discrimination.
- Although this patient does not mean to cause offence by his remarks, to ignore his use of these derogatory terms could be interpreted as tacit acceptance of his inappropriate language.
- The doctor–patient relationship is usually one based on trust and involves a duty of care on the doctor towards the patient. This can make it difficult to confront patients over inappropriate or offensive behaviour or language. However, as healthcare professionals, we need to uphold high standards and ensure that the environment we work in is free from discriminatory terminology or practices.
- You can allow him to finish his opening narrative, then explain that the words he has used are considered offensive and ask him not to use them again.
- How you deliver this comment is key – be polite but clear in your request – e.g. *"Some people find the words you use to describe the Chinese meal and the shop run by British Asians offensive. Can I ask you not to repeat them? Thank you."*
- If the patient responds in a hostile way, then you will need to deal with his anger before moving on (see Examination 2: Station 9).
- When possible, move the patient on by asking about his physical complaint, demonstrating a caring and professional consulting style, and treating him in just the same way as you would any other patient.

Domain 2 – Data gathering, examination and clinical assessment skills

History taking skills

You need to take an appropriate history to exclude red flags and to try and understand the impact of the patient's symptoms on his daily life:

- He says that his indigestion has got worse recently, can he say more about this?
- How long has he suffered from this problem?
- Can he tell you more about his indigestion – what does it feel like? Does he ever get the sensation of acid coming up into his mouth? Is it worse lying down?
- Where exactly does he feel the discomfort? Does it radiate anywhere, e.g. through to his back or into his arms?
- How bad have things been at their worst?
- He says that take-away foods make things worse – does anything else bring on his indigestion? What helps relieve his symptoms?
- Does he have the discomfort constantly or intermittently? What are things like at night?
- Has he felt nauseous or vomited?
- Any bleeding from his back passage? Have his stools become darker or appeared tarry black?
- Has he lost any weight recently? What is his appetite like?
- Any difficulty swallowing?
- Any chest pain when he exerts himself? Does he ever get short of breath with the indigestion pain?
- Does he smoke? How much alcohol does he drink?
- What sort of impact are his symptoms having on his day-to-day life? Has he had to take time off work due to his problem?
- Has he been under particular stress recently?
- You know that he is prescribed amlodipine for hypertension. Does he use this regularly and does he take any other medication, including over-the-counter drugs, such as ibuprofen? See Knowledge-base for information on drugs that can cause dyspepsia.
- What does he think is going on with his worsening symptoms? What is he hoping will come from seeing you today?

Physical examination skills

This is a fairly full station, with candidates needing to cover the issues around the patient's language, his presentation with dyspepsia, and management of his symptoms, including lifestyle advice, all in 10 min. You should say that you would like to examine his abdomen, but you will be told the findings and not be required actually to perform the examination:

The only positive findings on abdominal examination are obesity and mild tenderness on deep palpation of the epigastrium.

Domain 3 – Clinical management skills

Reaching a shared management plan (overlap with Domain 1)

This patient's diagnosis is uninvestigated dyspepsia with no red flag symptoms or signs. Given his age, history and examination findings, there is currently no indication for endoscopy (see Knowledge-base). If you decide to prescribe for dyspepsia, note that the GP curriculum states that you should be able to demonstrate a consistent and evidence-based approach:

- Reassure the patient that his symptoms are common and that there are no worrying signs.
- Empathize with him that dyspepsia can be very unpleasant and that you understand how it is now significantly affecting his quality of life.
- Explain that lifestyle changes could help his symptoms considerably, including:
  - Stopping smoking
  - Cutting down on alcohol
  - Losing weight.
- What small steps might he realistically be able to take, to start to make these changes?
- Other measures that he may find helpful include:
  - Raising the head of his bed
  - Avoiding eating late in the evening
  - Cutting down on spicy and fatty foods
  - Cutting down on caffeine and chocolate.
- Discuss how the medication he takes for his blood pressure might be making his symptoms worse, and that one option is to change to another tablet. What does he think about this?
- Other options which you could discuss with him include:
  - Empirical treatment with a proton pump inhibitor (PPI) for 1 month – e.g. omeprazole 20 mg OD or lansoprazole 30 mg OD.
  - Testing for *Helicobacter pylori* – using either urea breath test, stool antigen test or laboratory-based serology (if locally validated), and treating if appropriate.
- NICE states that there is no strong evidence as to which of the above two options (trial of a PPI or *Helicobacter pylori* test and treat) should be tried first.
- However, the patient is keen for you to prescribe him something to help with his symptoms, so a trial of a PPI with a review in a month might be the most appropriate option, so long as you make it clear that this should be in addition to lifestyle changes.
- Explain that if the trial of a PPI together with lifestyle changes helps to control his symptoms, then he should try and return to self-treatment with antacid and/or alginate therapy, as required.
- Make sure you safety-net appropriately – explain that the patient should seek immediate medical help if he experiences any signs or symptoms suggesting a perforation or gastrointestinal bleed.

Knowledge-base

National Institute for Clinical Excellence (NICE) (2004). CG 17 Dyspepsia – management of dyspepsia in adults in primary care (Quick Reference Guide). London: NICE. www.nice.org.uk/CG017. Reproduced with permission.

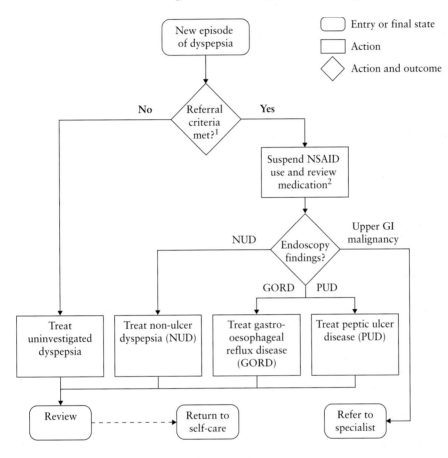

[1]Immediate referral is indicated for significant acute GI bleeding. Consider the possibility of cardiac or biliary disease as part of the differential diagnosis. Urgent specialist referral (i.e. within 2 weeks) for endoscopic investigation is indicated for patients of any age with dyspepsia when presenting with any of the following: chronic gastrointestinal bleeding, progressive unintentional weight loss, progressive difficulty swallowing, persistent vomiting, iron deficiency anaemia, epigastric mass or suspicious barium meal. Routine endoscopic investigation of patients of any age, presenting with dyspepsia and without alarm signs, is not necessary. However, in patients aged 55 years and older with unexplained [*can be taken to mean that common precipitants, such as NSAIDs, have been excluded; see NICE guidelines for full definition*] and persistent [*can be taken to mean up to 4–6 weeks, depending on the signs and symptoms; see NICE guidelines for full definition*] recent-onset dyspepsia alone, an urgent referral for endoscopy should be made.

[2]Review medications for possible causes of dyspepsia, e.g. calcium antagonists, nitrates, theophyllines, bisphosphonates, steroids and NSAIDs. Patients undergoing endoscopy should be free from medication with either a proton pump inhibitor (PPI) or an H_2 receptor antagonist (H_2RA) for a minimum of 2 weeks.

Take home messages

- We all have a duty to challenge discriminatory language or behaviour by patients or colleagues.
- Endoscopy is not routinely indicated for patients presenting with dyspepsia.
- The management of uninvestigated dyspepsia in primary care includes modifying exacerbating factors, lifestyle advice, trial of a PPI and *H. pylori* testing.

Ideas for further revision

Try role-playing with colleagues what you would say to patients who: made derogatory comments about another GP at your practice; swore at you during the consultation; or made sexually inappropriate comments about one of the reception staff.

Further reading

Delaney BC. 10-minute consultation: Dyspepsia. *BMJ* 2001;**322**:776. www.bmj.com.

Jankowski J, Jones R, Delaney B, Dent J. 10-minute consultation: Gastro-oesophageal reflux disease. *BMJ* 2002;**325**:945. www.bmj.com.

MeReC Briefing: The management of dyspepsia in primary care. March 2005. Issues no. 32. Pages 1–8. www.npc.co.uk/MeReC_Briefings/2006/dyspepsia_briefing_no_32.pdf.

NICE guidelines: Dyspepsia – management of dyspepsia in adults in primary care. August 2004 (amended June 2005). www.nice.org.uk.

RCGP curriculum statement 15.2 – Clinical Management: Digestive problems. www.rcgp.org.uk.

Information given to candidates

Mary French is a 48-year-old patient who suffers from hypertension.

Her blood pressure has been well controlled, with the most recent readings being:

128/82 – last week
126/76 – last month
132/78 – 6 months ago

She has been taking lisinopril 10 mg OD for 3 years without any problems.

Cervical smears – up to date and normal.

Height – 152 cm; weight – 53 kg; BMI – 23 kg/m²

Her records show that she is a nurse who works in the local gynaecology out-patient department.

Recent blood test results which the patient asked a colleague to take at work:

FBC	Normal	Glucose	Normal
U&Es	Normal	Total cholesterol	3.0 mmol/L
LFTs	Normal	HDL	1.6 mmol/L
TFTs	Normal	LDL	1.4 mmol/L
FSH	40 IU/L		
LH	20 IU/L		

As the patient enters the room she says, "Doctor, I think I'm going through the change and I really need something for my hot flushes and sweats – I know that there's an increased risk of breast cancer, DVTs and PEs, but do you think HRT would help?"

- What do you think this station is testing?
- Make notes or discuss your thoughts with a colleague before you read on.

Plan your approach to this station:

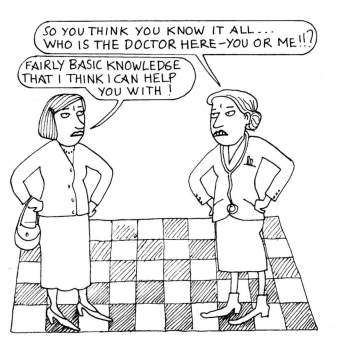

Information given to simulated patient

Basic details – You are Mary French, a Caucasian 48-year-old nurse.

Appearance and behaviour – You come across as confident and fairly knowledgeable about hormone replacement therapy (HRT). You occasionally use medical jargon such as 'perimenopausal' (meaning around the time of the menopause) and 'PE' (pulmonary embolism – a blood clot in the lung).

History

Freely divulged to doctor – Your periods used to be 'like clockwork' but over the last 9 months they have become more and more irregular. You now have a period every 2–3 months. You have been suffering from worsening hot flushes and night sweats for the last 12 months. These really bother you, particularly at work and in the summer. You know about HRT through your work, and you also had an informal chat with one of the gynaecology doctors about whether you should start HRT. She talked about some of the risks and benefits but said that you should discuss things with your GP. You have read that there is a 50% increased risk of breast cancer with HRT and want to discuss this with the doctor.

Divulged to doctor if specifically asked – You or your immediate family have never had any problems with clots in your limbs or lungs. You do not suffer from varicose veins. You have never had any gynaecological problems or operations. You do not have migraines or diabetes. You have never had any heart problems and the nurse said that your recent cholesterol test was 'very good'. Your great aunt was diagnosed with breast cancer when she was in her 80s, but died of a stroke soon thereafter. You used to have a coil fitted for contraception but for the last 5 years have been using condoms with your husband. You have not experienced any problems with vaginal dryness or urinary symptoms. Your mood has been fine.

Ideas, concerns and expectations – You are aware of the 'media scares' about HRT being associated with breast cancer and blood clots and, despite your work, you still feel a little anxious about starting HRT. In particular, you are concerned that your great aunt had breast cancer, and that you used to smoke and now have tablets for blood pressure. You are unsure to what degree these factors could further increase the risks of taking HRT. From the knowledge you have already, and because your symptoms are so unpleasant, you have rationalized that you should probably try HRT but you want the doctor to go over the risks and hopefully reassure you that these are small. Your friend has HRT patches and you know how to use these, and if you decide to start HRT today, then you would like to try patches first. You also want to know what the doctor thinks about herbal alternatives.

First words spoken to doctor – "Doctor, I think I'm going through the change and I really need something for my hot flushes and sweats – I know that there's an increased risk of breast cancer, DVTs and PEs, but do you think HRT would help?"

Past medical history – You were diagnosed with high blood pressure 3 years ago and this has been well controlled with medication.

Drug history – You take one lisinopril 10 mg tablet every morning. You are not allergic to any medication.

Social history – You work at the local hospital in the gynaecology outpatient department. You also work the occasional evening shift at a family planning clinic. You live with your husband and have one grown up daughter who lives abroad. You smoked about five cigarettes a day from when you were aged 18–22. You drink the odd gin and tonic if you go out at the weekend. You attend two step-aerobic classes every week.

Family history – There are no major health problems in your immediate family.

- Having read the information given to the simulated patient, what do you now think this station is testing?
- Make notes or discuss your thoughts with a colleague before you turn the page.

Review your approach to this station:

Tested at this station:

1. History taking skills
2. Communicating risk
3. Reaching a shared management plan with an expert patient

Domain 2 – Data gathering, examination and clinical assessment skills

History taking skills

This patient is asking about HRT as a means to control her perimenopausal symptoms. Before you discuss the pros and cons of treatment, you need to take a careful history to help assess whether HRT would be suitable in her case. Always remember to start with open questions and elicit the patient's ideas, concerns and expectations, before narrowing the focus of the history to specific closed questions:

- The patient thinks that she is 'going through the change' – can she say more about this? What symptoms is she experiencing? What is happening with her periods?
- She mentions HRT – what does she know about this treatment? What are her thoughts about HRT?
- She talks about the increased risk of breast cancer, DVTs and PEs with HRT – can she say more about this? What are her particular concerns?
- Does she smoke?
- Has she or any member of her immediate family ever had a deep vein thrombosis (DVT) – *'a blood clot usually in the leg or arm'* or a pulmonary embolus (PE) – *'a blood clot in the lung'*? Although the patient has used these acronyms, it is important to be clear exactly what you mean by them.
- Has she ever had any problems with lumps in her breasts or any abnormality on breast screening (mammography)?
- Has she ever had any gynaecological problems – such as endometriosis?
- Has she ever had any gynaecological surgery – in particular, does she still have a womb?
- Does she suffer from varicose veins or migraines?
- Does she have any other medical problems, such as diabetes or heart problems?
- How has her mood been?
- How are her symptoms affecting her work and home life? Who else is at home with her?
- What was she hoping would happen from coming to the surgery today?

Domain 1 – Interpersonal skills

Communicating risk

This patient already knows that there are some added risks in taking HRT, but she is keen for you to explain these fully, and hopefully reassure her that the risks are small:

- Communicating risk in terms that patients can readily understand can be a challenge to health professionals.
- Suggestions to facilitate understanding include describing absolute risk rather than relative risk – i.e. *"The risk increases from 1 in a 1000 to 2 in a 1000"* rather than *"The risk increases by 100%"*.
- She mentions the increased risk of breast cancer, DVTs and PEs with HRT. Does she also know about the small increased risk of stroke, endometrial cancer and ovarian cancer (the latter two in those using oestrogen-only HRT)?
- The patient is concerned about her blood pressure and previous smoking. You could reassure her that she has only accumulated one pack year of smoking, over 25 years ago, which is unlikely to have a significant effect on the risks associated with HRT.
- Her blood pressure has been well controlled since diagnosis, her cholesterol level is low and she has no history of heart problems. You could inform her that, although the product literature advises caution in prescribing HRT to patients with hypertension, the BNF states that evidence for this advice is unsatisfactory and many women with such a diagnosis may stand to benefit from HRT. However, it would be important for her to continue having her blood pressure monitored regularly. What does she think about this?
- She has specifically referred to the risks of breast cancer and thromboembolism. Would she like more detailed information on these risks?
- If so, you could go through the introductory section on HRT in the BNF together, explaining that about 14 in every 1000 women aged 50–64 years not using HRT have breast cancer diagnosed over 5 years, whereas in those taking HRT for 5 years there are about six extra cases per 1000 women.
- This patient had a great aunt who developed breast cancer in her 80s. One of the cautions for use of HRT is having risk factors for oestrogen-dependent tumours – such as breast cancer in a first-degree relative. Hence, only having a third-degree relative with breast cancer should not be a reason for caution. (See NICE guidelines in Further reading for information on family history and breast cancer risk.)
- Similarly you could go through the increased risks of thromboembolism on HRT (see Knowledge-base).
- Does she understand what the figures mean in terms of small increased risks?
- Would she like written material to take away with her?
- She wants to know what you think about herbal alternatives to HRT. You could advise her that the evidence for their use is conflicting and that some can interact with prescription medications. There is also the concern regarding the quality and quantity of active ingredient in some products marketed as herbal alternatives to HRT.
- You have discussed the risks with her in some detail. Remember to advise her of the proven benefits of HRT in terms of symptomatic relief – of particular importance to her – and osteoporosis protection, together with a reduced risk of colorectal cancer (see Knowledge-base).

Domain 3 – Clinical management skills

Reaching a shared management plan with an expert patient

Mrs French is an 'expert' patient in that, through her work, she already knows about indications and some of the risk factors for HRT, plus she has discussed her situation informally with a specialist medical colleague. You need to acknowledge and respond to her level of knowledge and ensure that you will involve her fully in a jointly agreed management plan:

- It can sometimes feel challenging dealing with well informed patients. Indeed, some expert patients will know more about their medical condition than their GP. The key here is not to see such patients as a threat, but as an opportunity for full patient involvement in the management – including self-management – of their condition, and as a chance for health professional education too.
- Start with general advice about lifestyle measures that may help with symptoms, such as avoiding triggers – e.g. caffeine, alcohol or certain foods – and wearing loose fitting, cotton clothes. To slow bone loss, encourage regular weight-bearing exercise – this patient already attends aerobic classes twice a week.
- Having taken a thorough history and determined that there are no contraindications to the patient having HRT, and after discussing the risks and benefits of HRT fully with the patient, what are her thoughts about this treatment option?
- Explain that there are other prescribed medication alternatives to HRT (see Knowledge-base) but that these are not optimal treatments and are usually considered when women cannot or do not want to take HRT.
- As she may know, options for using HRT include tablets, patches, implants, gels and vaginal rings. She has expressed an interest in patches, which you could offer to prescribe.
- Is she aware that HRT does not provide contraception and that women < 50 years are considered potentially fertile for up to 2 years after their last menstrual period (and for those aged > 50, for 1 year after their last menstrual period)? Is she happy with the current method of contraception she and her husband are using?
- Advise the patient that she should stop taking HRT and seek urgent medical help if she experiences any of the following:
  - Sudden severe chest pain or shortness of breath
  - Cough with blood-stained sputum
  - Unexplained severe pain in the calf of one leg
  - Serious neurological symptoms such as severe and prolonged headache, loss of vision, or weakness or numbness affecting one part of her body.
- Side effects she might experience from HRT include: fluid retention, breast tenderness, headaches, breakthrough bleeding, weight gain and bloating.
- Arrange to review her in 3 months, or sooner if any problems develop.

Knowledge-base – HRT

References – BNF, NHS Clinical Knowledge Summaries.

Hormone replacement therapy (HRT)	*Options*: • Small dose of an oestrogen • Plus a progestogen if intact uterus • Tibolone (some androgenic action)	*Alternatives to HRT for symptomatic relief*: • Herbal remedies (conflicting evidence of effectiveness) • Clonidine (poor side effect profile) • Antidepressants – e.g. fluoxetine, paroxetine, citalopram and venlafaxine • Gabapentin
Pros/cons of HRT	*Pros*: • Alleviates menopausal symptoms – e.g. vaginal dryness and vasomotor instability (hot flushes, sweats) • ↓ Postmenopausal osteoporosis, but should not be used solely for this purpose • ↓ Risk of colorectal cancer	*Cons*: • ↑ Risk of thromboembolism • ↑ Risk of stroke • ↑ Risk of breast cancer • ↑ Risk of endometrial cancer in those using oestrogen-only HRT • ↑ Risk of ovarian cancer in those using oestrogen-only HRT
Management	• Treatment advised at minimum effective dose for the shortest duration • Review annually • For osteoporosis, consider alternative treatments	• Should not be used to protect against cognitive function – no indication • Should not be used to prevent CHD – no indication. Indeed, may ↑ risk in the first year of treatment • Experience limited with women > 65 years
Risk of breast cancer	• All types of HRT ↑ risk of breast cancer within 1–2 years of starting treatment • ↑ Risk related to duration of treatment • ↑ Risk not related to age when starting treatment • Excess risk gone within approximately 5 years of stopping	• Baseline – about 14 in every 1000 women aged 50–64 years *not* using HRT have breast cancer diagnosed over 5 years • Combined HRT for 5 years = about 6 *extra* cases per 1000 women • Oestrogen-only HRT for 5 years = about 1.5 *extra* cases per 1000 women • Tibolone ↑ risk of breast cancer but to a lesser extent than combined HRT
Risk of DVT/PE	• Combined or oestrogen-only HRT ↑ risk of DVT and PE especially in first year of treatment • If predisposing factors present – personal or family history of DVT/PE, severe varicose veins, obesity, trauma, or prolonged bed-rest – review need for HRT as risks may outweigh benefits	• Baseline – about 10 in every 1000 women aged 50–59 years *not* using HRT develop venous thromboembolism over 5 years • Combined HRT for 5 years = about 4 *extra* cases per 1000 women • Oestrogen-only HRT for 5 years = about 1 *extra* case per 1000 women

Cautions and contraindications	Contraindications: • Oestrogen-dependent cancer • History of breast cancer • Pregnancy or breast feeding • Active thrombophlebitis • Angina or myocardial infarction • Deep vein thrombosis or recurrent thromboembolism (unless anticoagulated) • Liver disease	Cautions: • Prolonged exposure to unopposed oestrogen may ↑ risk of endometrial cancer • History of breast nodules or fibrocystic disease • Breast cancer in first-degree relative • Factors ↑ risk of thromboembolism • Migraine • Diabetes (increased risk of heart disease)

Take home messages

- For the treatment of menopausal symptoms the benefits of short-term HRT outweigh the risks for the majority of women.
- Explaining risks to patients in terms they can understand is a skill which can be readily assessed in the CSA.
- A consultation with an expert patient should be seen as an opportunity for full patient participation.

Ideas for further revision

Make sure you are able to explain the risks and benefits associated with a range of interventions in primary care, such as prescribing combined and progestogen-only hormonal contraceptives, HRT, aspirin and steroid use, together with the pros and cons of undertaking certain tests, such as the prostate-specific antigen (PSA) test.

Further reading

British Menopause Society Council consensus statement on hormone replacement therapy 2006. www.thebms.org.uk/statementcontent.php?id=1.

British National Formulary (BNF). Published jointly by BMJ Publishing Group and RPS Publishing, London. Updated every 6 months. www.bnf.org.

Menopause Matters – an independent, clinician-led website. www.menopausematters.co.uk.

Million Women Study Collaborators. Breast cancer and hormone replacement therapy in the Million Women Study. *Lancet* 2003;**362**:419–427.

NHS National Library for Health Clinical Knowledge Summaries – 1. Hormone replacement therapy 2. Breast cancer – managing women with a family history. www.cks.library.nhs.uk/clinical_knowledge.

NICE guideline on familial breast cancer. (Guideline no. 14) 2004. www.nice. org.uk/pdf/CG014niceguideline.pdf.

RCGP curriculum statement 10.1 – Women's health. www.rcgp.org.uk.

Women's Health Initiative Study. www.whi.org.

Information given to candidates

Barry Southgate is a 20 year old who has recently registered at your practice.

Last week he saw the practice nurse for a new patient check and told her that he has been taking heroin for 18 months, but now wants to 'kick the habit'.

The nurse noted:

Smoker	10 roll-up cigarettes a day
Alcohol	Rarely
Height	170 cm
Weight	51 kg
BMI	17.6 kg/m^2
Urinalysis	Normal
BP	126/72

Your practice has a shared-care arrangement with the local specialist addiction unit. One of your GP colleagues, Dr Black, together with support from the local drugs service, runs a weekly clinic in the GP surgery, in which opiate replacement treatment is routinely prescribed.

As the patient walks into the consultation room he says, "I really want to get off the heroin, and need your help doc."

- What do you think this station is testing?
- Make notes or discuss your thoughts with a colleague before you read on.

Plan your approach to this station:

Information given to simulated patient

Basic details – You are Barry Southgate, a Caucasian 20-year-old former labourer.

Appearance and behaviour – You are a little agitated and fidgety during the consultation. You are underweight. You make good eye contact and are casually dressed in clothes that are overdue for a change.

History

Freely divulged to doctor – You have been using heroin continuously for about 18 months, at first smoking and then injecting. You have never sought help for this before. You thought you were in control of things, but having lost your job and split up with your partner because of your drug use, you realize that you need help. You are hoping that the doctor can prescribe you some methadone today.

Divulged to doctor if specifically asked – To begin with you were funding your drug use from your wages and by borrowing money, but since you lost your job 1 year ago you have been shop-lifting as a source of money to buy drugs. You have been cautioned by the police, but have never been to prison. You have not been to hospital as the result of an overdose or any other drug-related problem. Over the last 4 months you have started occasionally injecting into your groin, as you find it increasingly difficult to find veins elsewhere in your arms or legs. You shared needles with your brother on several occasions. You have not been tested or vaccinated for hepatitis or HIV.

Ideas, concerns and expectations – Two weeks ago one of your friends had an overdose when injecting heroin after being released from prison. You were with him when this happened. You called 999 but were scared that the police might be involved, so you did not stay for the ambulance. You have heard that he is OK, but this incident has made you think about your own drug use – you are worried that the same thing could happen to you and want to get help to tackle your problem. Initially you will be annoyed if the doctor says that you cannot start methadone today. However, if the doctor explains why this is the case, and is understanding of your circumstances, then you will agree to come to the dedicated clinic at the surgery. You will be happy to accept any offers of testing for HIV or hepatitis, and hepatitis vaccinations, which you have been meaning to have done for some time. You do not want to think about seeking help from housing or welfare projects yet, until you are more stable on methadone and off heroin.

First words spoken to doctor – "I really want to get off the heroin, and need your help doc."

Past medical history – You have never had any problems with infected injection sites or abscesses. You have not had any blood clots in your limbs or lungs. You have lost nearly 3 stones in weight over the last year, as you often go without meals. Your teeth have been giving you trouble lately, but the heroin helps with the pain. You were fit and well before you started taking heroin.

Drug history – You are currently using two to three £10 bags of heroin a day, injecting three times a day. About twice a week you smoke crack cocaine and you use cannabis to help 'come down' from the crack. Before you first tried heroin you used to take speed (amphetamines) and ecstasy. As far as you know, you are not allergic to any medication.

Social history – You split up with your partner 6 months ago, after repeatedly arguing about your drug use, and have been staying with various friends since then. You do not have any children. You have spent the odd night sleeping on the streets when you could not find accommodation. Your mother has said that she won't speak to you again until you are drug-free as you started to steal from her to fund your heroin use. You smoke about 10 roll-up cigarettes a day. You hardly ever drink alcohol. You have not worked for the last year, ever since your heroin use got out of control and you were sacked for being off sick regularly. You do not drive.

Family history – Your father died of alcohol-related liver problems in his 50s. You have one brother who is currently in prison for burglary. He has had a blood clot in his leg through injecting into his groin.

- Having read the information given to the simulated patient, what do you now think this station is testing?
- Make notes or discuss your thoughts with a colleague before you turn the page.

Review your approach to this station:

Tested at this station:

1. Ability to engage constructively with a patient who misuses drugs
2. Taking a drug misuse history
3. Recognizing limits of competence
4. Management of first presentation of drug misuse

Domain 1 – Interpersonal skills

Ability to engage constructively with a patient who misuses drugs

The most important goal with patients who misuse drugs is to try and engender a sense of trust and hope, so that they will engage with services and return to see you for follow-up care:

- Be empathetic and find out about the patient's agenda – what are his ideas, concerns and expectations from coming to see you today?
- Drug-using patients have the right to access good quality services. You must demonstrate a non-judgemental approach and not let any personal opinion of a perceived self-inflicted problem affect his care.
- Encourage hope – positively affirm his actions in taking the important first step to address his drug use by coming down to the surgery today.
- Explain that change is not easy and that he may have relapses along the way, but the important thing is that he is motivated and wants to change.
- Explain that prescribing methadone – or any equivalent opiate replacement medication – is only one part of a package of care that needs to be put in place to help support him, once a full assessment has been done.

Domain 2 – Data gathering, examination and clinical assessment skills

Taking a drug misuse history

You need to tailor your history to cover the pertinent issues surrounding the patient's drug misuse:

- Start with open questions – can he tell you more about his drug use? What impact has it had on his life?
- More specific questions which may help give a detailed picture of the patient's drug use include:
    1. *Drugs*:
        - What drugs does he use? How much of each does he use? How long has he been using each one?
        - Remember also specifically to ask about cannabis and alcohol use, as these are often not seen as relevant by patients who misuse drugs.
        - Does he inject or smoke each drug? If he injects, does he ever share needles or injecting equipment? Where does he inject?
        - How much does he use of each drug each day, or per week? Where does he get the drugs from?
        - Does he take the drugs on his own or with others?

2. *Treatment*:
   ○ Any previous treatment for his drug use?
   ○ Has he had any periods of being drug-free since he started?
3. *Physical and mental problems:*
   ○ Any physical problems as a result of his drug use, such as clots, abscesses or infections? Has he ever had a drug overdose?
   ○ Does he suffer from asthma? Inhaled drugs and stimulants can exacerbate asthma.
   ○ Any time in hospital as a result of his drug use?
   ○ Any mental health problems, such as depression or self-harm? Has he ever seen a mental health specialist such as a psychiatrist?
4. *Forensic history:*
   ○ Has he ever been involved with the criminal justice system as a result of his drug use? – e.g. time in prison or on a community drugs order, or on probation.
   ○ Are there any court cases pending? Being engaged with drugs services may help with sentencing and could be a reason for presenting now.
5. *Vaccinations and testing:*
   ○ Has he had any blood tests for viruses like hepatitis or HIV?
   ○ Has he been vaccinated for hepatitis? Can he remember which type – A or B? What about tetanus vaccination?
6. *Social situation:*
   ○ Where is he living at the moment? Has he ever been homeless as a result of his drug use?
   ○ Does he have a partner? Are there any children living with him or visiting regularly?
   ○ Is he working?
● Remember – the list above is only a guide – it is more important that you respond to the patient's agenda and concerns, and demonstrate an empathetic and understanding approach, rather than simply go through a checklist of questions.

Physical examination

When a drug user first presents it is good practice to examine him for evidence of drug use – e.g. needle track marks – and also to make sure that he has no problems like abscesses or a deep vein thrombosis (DVT). Are there any signs of intoxication today? You should also assess his mental state – is the patient depressed? Does he represent a suicide risk? At this station you will not have to physically examine the patient. However, you would be expected to attempt to examine him, at which point the examiner will tell you the findings – namely that there are needle track marks on the patient's arms and that he is thin, but that otherwise examination is normal.

Domain 3 – Clinical management skills

Recognizing limits of competence

The Department of Health guidelines (see Further reading) make clear that all doctors should be equipped to deal with drug-related issues. However, for the GP inexperienced in dealing with patients who misuse drugs, this might mean appropriate support, advice and general medical care, plus referral to a GP colleague or the local specialist drugs service for further management:

- Acknowledge his desire to start medication straight away, but explain that your practice works in partnership with the local specialist drugs service in offering a dedicated clinic once a week, here at the surgery, at which your colleague, Dr Black can prescribe opiate replacement treatment, such as methadone, if this is appropriate. Do not feel pressurized by the patient into prescribing outside the limits of your competence.
- Explain that there is still much that you can help with today, and that at the end of the consultation you could help book an appointment for him at Dr Black's next clinic.
- It is far better in the first consultation with a drug user to show empathy and support, and make clear that the patient's needs will be addressed, than be rushed into prescribing before a full and proper assessment has been undertaken.

Management of first presentation of drug misuse

There is much that you can offer a patient who first presents with problem drug use. But remember that you only have 10 min for the station, so you need to be focused:

- Despite not being in a position to prescribe opiate replacement treatment to the patient today, you should still:
  - Offer basic harm minimization advice and health promotion – e.g.:
    - Safer injecting advice – not to share; use clean needles; avoid the groin or neck; not to inject on own
    - Needle exchange information
    - Sexual health advice – e.g. encourage condom use
    - Screening for blood-borne viruses (hepatitis B, C and HIV).
  - Offer hepatitis A and B, plus tetanus vaccination. The RCGP guidelines (see Further reading) recommend opportunistic vaccination, rather than waiting to check serology first.
  - Offer general medical care – e.g. smoking cessation advice, dietary advice.
  - Signpost him to other services – e.g.:
    - Citizen's Advice Bureau for benefits advice
    - Local authority or homelessness project for housing advice
    - Local NHS dentist for an assessment.
- You could explain that before opiate replacement treatment – such as methadone – is prescribed, it is usual for a urine sample to be taken to confirm opiate use. You could offer to take a sample now and send it off for toxicology, as this might help speed things up when he attends Dr Black's clinic.
- You are expected to report when drug misusers first present for treatment – or re-present after a gap of 6 months or more – to the regional or national drug misuse database. For more details see the British National Formulary (BNF) section in Further reading.

Knowledge-base – Management of drug misuse

Reference – GP curriculum statement 15.3, citing *Task Force to Review Services for Drug Misusers* – see Further reading.

Hierarchy of goals of drug treatment

Abstinence from all drugs

Abstinence from main problem drugs

Attainment of controlled, non-dependent or non-problematical drug use

Reduction of health, social or other problems not directly attributable to drug misuse

Reduction of harmful or risky behaviours associated with the misuse of drugs – e.g. sharing injecting equipment

Reduction of health, social and other problems directly related to drug misuse

Take home messages

- Drug-using patients have complex problems and you should try and address their social, psychological and physical needs.
- You should only prescribe for drug misuse within the limits of your competence, and refer to GP colleagues with appropriate training or specialist centres for further management.
- There is still much that you can do to help drug-using patients presenting in primary care.

Ideas for further revision

The GP curriculum statement on drug and alcohol problems suggests that GP specialty registrars should be encouraged to look after some of their practice's drug-using patients and follow them through their patient journey. In addition, you may find the interactive RCGP e-learning modules on substance misuse helpful (see Further reading).

Further reading

Beaumont B (ed). *Care of Drug Users in General Practice,* 2nd edn. Oxford: Radcliffe Publishing, 2004.

British Medical Association and Royal Pharmaceutical Society of Great Britain. *The British National Formulary 53* Section: Guidance of prescribing – Controlled drugs and drug dependence; notification of drug misusers. London: BMJ Books, 2007. www.bnf.org.uk.

Department of Health, Scottish Office Home and Health Department, Welsh Office. *Drug Misuse and Dependence, Guidelines on Clinical Management.* London: The Stationery Office, 1999. (Note: Draft of updated guidelines is out for consultation in 2007.)

Drugs.gov.uk. Latest government policy, research, legislation, good practice and guidance. www.drugs.gov.uk.

National Institute of Health and Clinical Excellence. *Drug misuse: opioid detoxification.* London: NICE, 2007. www.nice.org.uk/CG0512.

NHS National Library for Health Clinical Knowledge Summaries – Opioid dependence. www.cks.library.nhs.uk/clinical_knowledge.

RCGP curriculum statement 15.3 – Clinical Management: Drug and alcohol problems. www.rcgp.org.uk.

RCGP substance misuse interactive e-learning modules (forms part of RCGP Certificate in the Management of Drug Misuse part 1). www.rcgp.org.uk/substance_misuse/substance_misuse_home/elearning.aspx.

Royal College of General Practitioners. *Guidance for hepatitis A and B vaccination of drug users in primary care and criteria for audit.* London: RCGP, 2005. www.rcgp.org.uk/PDF/drug_hepAB.pdf.

Substance Misuse Management in General Practice. The GP curriculum statement recommends this as the best website for GPs on drug misuse. www.smmgp.org.uk.

Task Force to Review Services for Drug Misusers. *Report of an Independent Survey of Drug Treatment Services in England.* London: Department of Health, 1996.

Information given to candidates

Johan Slemick is a 72-year-old retired insurance broker.

He saw your GP colleague – Dr Umesh – 10 days ago with a history of haemoptysis, worsening cough and weight loss.

He has smoked 20 cigarettes a day for 50 years.

The patient's notes state that he has COPD and is prescribed:

- Salbutamol metered dose inhaler (MDI) 100 μg – two puffs BD
- Tiotropium 18 μg (one dry powder inhalation) OD
- Salmeterol MDI 25 μg – two puffs BD
- Aspirin 75 mg OD

Examination 10 days ago revealed reduced air entry at the right lung base.

Dr Umesh requested an urgent chest X-ray and asked the patient to return to discuss the findings.

The chest X-ray report reads:

'There is a large (3 cm diameter) suspicious-looking shadow in the right hilar area. The lungs are hyper-expanded, consistent with a diagnosis of COPD. Given the patient's smoking history and current symptoms, there is a high probability of neoplastic pathology. Suggest referral for urgent bronchoscopy.'

Dr Umesh is on holiday this week so the patient has been booked in with you.

As the patient enters the room he says, "Hello doctor, I got a call asking me to come in to discuss my chest X-ray result."

- What do you think this station is testing?
- Make notes or discuss your thoughts with a colleague before you read on.

Plan your approach to this station:

Information given to simulated patient

Basic details – You are Johan Slemick, a Caucasian 72-year-old retired insurance broker.

Appearance and behaviour – At first you appear relaxed and confident. However, when the doctor tells you the chest X-ray result you are initially distressed (despite having suspected that it might be something serious – see Ideas, concerns and expectations).

History

Freely divulged to doctor – You had been meaning to come to the doctor's for some time as your cough has been getting worse over the last 2–3 months. Then, 10 days ago, you coughed up bright fresh blood. You have never coughed up blood before, so you came straight down to the surgery. The doctor examined you and arranged for a chest X-ray. Yesterday you had one more episode of coughing up blood. As before, this was a small to medium amount of bright red blood.

Divulged to doctor if specifically asked – You have lost about one and a half stones in weight over the last few months, but as you were overweight to begin with you thought that this could only be a good thing. Your appetite has been poor for the last month. You always suffered from a 'smoker's cough' and see the doctor for antibiotics for 'bronchitis' at least a couple of times a year. You have not had any chest infections recently, although you do feel a bit more 'out of puff'. You have not had any chest pain. If the doctor says that the X-ray suggests that things could be serious, you will ask directly if it is cancer. Despite usually being the sort of person who wants to know all about your health, today you will initially say – when told that it could be cancer – that you don't want to know any more details. But if the doctor appears kind and understanding, and asks more about your concerns, you will disclose your worries at this news, and agree to come back and see the doctor in a few days to discuss your options. You do not want to talk today about any more tests as you just want to 'get your head' round the possibility that it could be very serious. You do not want your wife told at this stage.

Ideas, concerns and expectations – When you coughed up blood you started to feel uneasy about what was going on. You were hoping that it was due to the 'bronchitis'. Neither yourself nor the doctor you saw last time mentioned that it might be something serious, but it worried you that he marked the X-ray card 'Urgent'. It was then that you thought it might be cancer. An old work friend died from lung cancer a couple of years ago, and you remember that it had started with him coughing up blood. You have been trying to tell yourself that it's going to be OK, but deep down you feel less confident. All sorts of negative thoughts have been going through your mind, such as how your wife would cope if you became ill, and whether you will be well enough to go on the cruise you have booked for both of you in 4 months' time. You have been praying that the doctor would say today that the chest X-ray was fine and that it could all be put down to the 'bronchitis'.

First words spoken to doctor – "Hello doctor, I got a call asking me to come in to discuss my chest X-ray result."

Past medical history – For about 10 years you have been using inhalers to help with the damage done to your lungs through smoking. Otherwise you have been fairly healthy and have never had any serious illnesses.

Drug history – You have been using a blue inhaler (salbutamol), one or two puffs a couple of times a day, for about 10 years. A second inhaler, tiotropium, one inhalation once a day, was added 2 years ago, and last year your doctor also started you on a salmeterol inhaler – two puffs twice a day, to help with your worsening breathlessness. You are not allergic to any medication.

Social history – You have smoked since your early 20s – about 20 cigarettes a day. You have never seriously considered giving up smoking, as you 'really enjoy it'. You drink the occasional glass of wine with meals. You live with your wife, who has been suffering with her own health and mobility problems recently – last year she lost the sight in one eye due to a stroke and also fell and broke her hip. You were both looking forward to a month's cruise in the Caribbean in 4 months. You have a grown up son who lives in Spain.

Family history – There are no major health problems in your immediate family.

- Having read the information given to the simulated patient, what do you now think this station is testing?
- Make notes or discuss your thoughts with a colleague before you turn the page.

Review your approach to this station:

Tested at this station:

1. Breaking bad news
2. Negotiating with a patient regarding further management

Domains 1 and 2 – Interpersonal skills and Data gathering

Breaking bad news

Although there is no definite diagnosis at this stage, the chest X-ray result – together with the patient's history – is highly suspicious of a sinister pathology. You need to use skill and tact when breaking this bad news to the patient:

- Ask the patient to explain what first brought him to the surgery.
- Clarify events since he last saw your colleague.
- Explore his understanding of why the X-ray was requested.
- From his answers to the above, it should become clear whether the patient suspects a worrying finding. If not, then a more direct question would be useful – *"Have you thought about what the problem might be?"*
- Explore whether he is the type of person who likes to know all about his medical test results. Be careful not to impose information on a patient who gives verbal or non-verbal cues that he is reluctant to be told more.
- If the patient does appear to suspect something serious, then you need to explore in more detail his understanding about what the diagnosis could be.
- But if the patient appears not to have considered a serious pathology, then firing a warning shot will help in the process of breaking the bad news – e.g. *"I'm afraid the chest X-ray result is somewhat worrying"*.
- You may not have a firm diagnosis yet, but it is still important to explain the chest X-ray result fully and honestly, but without extinguishing hope.
- Give information in manageable chunks. Use pauses between chunks to allow the patient time to process his thoughts.
- Use silences to give the patient space to go at his own pace.
- Once you have disclosed the information about the chest X-ray findings, it is important to acknowledge and thereby give permission for any distress – e.g. *"I can see that you are very distressed at this news"*.
- Ask about the patient's concerns and feelings at the news.
- If he asks you directly whether it is cancer, do not side-step the question but explain that further tests would need to be done, but that lung cancer is a strong possibility.
- Again ask whether he has any further concerns. Do not move on to management options with a patient until you have elicited all the patient's concerns. In this case, he is particularly worried about what will happen to his wife if he becomes ill and whether he will be well enough to go on the upcoming cruise.
- Acknowledge that at this stage the diagnosis and prognosis are uncertain, and empathize at the distress this uncertainty itself may cause.

Domain 3 – Clinical management skills

Negotiating with a patient regarding further management

After breaking bad news and fully addressing the patient's concerns it is important to negotiate about how to proceed:

- Emphasize the fact that although the chest X-ray result is worrying, you will not have a firm diagnosis until further investigations are done.
- This patient does not want to discuss further tests today. Make sure you respect this and do not force information on him about bronchoscopy or referral to hospital.
- Explore why he feels this way and ask whether he would like to come back to see you again to discuss things further.
- Many patients, once they have heard that the diagnosis could be cancer, do not fully take in information about further tests or treatment options. So as well as respecting his views, it may also be useful to go over these at another appointment.
- Would he like to bring someone with him to the next appointment to provide support?
- You could also offer either to tell his wife, or to be present when he tells her, if he decides at some future point to discuss it with her.
- He may find it helpful to keep a note of any questions that come to him before seeing you again.
- How is he going to get home today? Is there anyone who could come to pick him up?

Knowledge-base – Breaking bad news

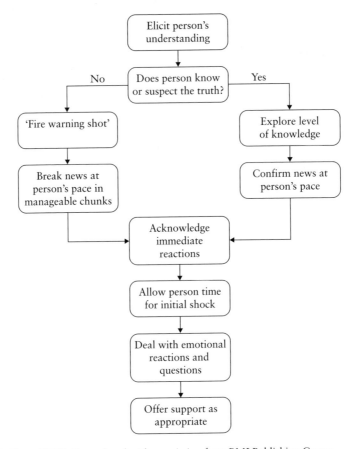

From Faulkner (1998). Reproduced with permission from BMJ Publishing Group.

Take home messages

- Never force information on patients unless they indicate that they want to know more.
- Breaking bad news can be emotionally draining for the doctor too. Debriefing with colleagues can help manage negative feelings generated by such consultations.

Ideas for further revision

Hospital posts that form part of GP specialty training programmes – such as A&E and elderly care – regularly require doctors to break bad news. You could first ask to sit in with an experienced, senior colleague. Then ask if they will sit in with you while you take the lead, and provide feedback on the consultation. Additionally, you could simulate such scenarios with peers or your trainer, or request formal sessions with fellow GP trainees using trained actors to take the patients' roles.

Further reading

Faulkner A. ABC of palliative care: Communication with patients, families, and other professionals. *BMJ* 1998;**316**:130–132. www.bmj.com.

Maguire P. *Communication Skills for Doctors*. London: Arnold, 2000: Chapter 6.

Mueller PS. Breaking bad news to patients – The SPIKES approach can make this difficult task easier. *Postgraduate Medicine Online*. September 2002;**112**(3). www.postgradmed.com/issues/2002/09_02/editorial_sep.htm.

RCGP curriculum statement 12 – Care of People with Cancer & Palliative Care. www.rcgp.org.uk.

Silverman J, Kurtz S, Draper J. *Skills for Communicating with Patients,* 2nd edn. Oxford: Radcliffe Medical Press, 2004.

Examination 1 – Grid of stations and clinical areas covered (categories taken from the core and extended statements of the new GP curriculum)

Category	1	2	3	4	5	6	7	8	9	10	11	12	13
Learn dis													
H Pro		×	×					×		×			
Drug use													
Psy	×				×			×					
Pall													
Sex					×					×			
M					×								
F											×		
Geri									×				
Paed			×										
Acute													
Gene													
Derm				×									
Rheum													×
Resp		×											
Neuro													
Endo							×						
Eye													
ENT						×				×			
GI												×	
CVD								×					

Case	Description
1	Depression; upset
2	Asthma; smoker
3	Mum re: obese son
4	Acne; wants Roaccutane
5	Erectile dysfunction
6	Otitis media; demanding
7	Complaint re colleague; diabetes
8	Hypertension
9	Dizziness
10	Glandular fever
11	Infertility
12	Crohn's disease; telephone
13	Back pain; talkative

Examination 1 – Primary nature of each case

Station	Gender mix	Age mix	Skills in diagnosis	Ongoing management skills	Clinical practical skills	Health promotion	Diversity and ethical issues	Dealing with patients' emotions
1 Depression	F	30						×
2 Asthma	M	54				×		
3 Obese son	F (mother)	44, son 11				×		
4 Acne	F	23		×				
5 Erectile dysfunction	M	54	×					
6 Ear infection	F	56						×
7 Complaint re colleague	F	48						×
8 Hypertension	M	58		×				
9 Dizziness	F	74			×			
10 Glandular fever	F	16	×					
11 Infertility	F	20	×					
12 Crohn's disease – telephone consultation	M	42		×				
13 Back pain	F	46			×			

Appendix 2

Examination 2 – Grid of stations and clinical areas covered (categories taken from the core and extended statements of the new GP curriculum)

	1	2	3	4	5	6	7	8	9	10	11	12	13
Learn dis			×										
H Pro												×	
Drug use												×	
Psy	×												
Pall													×
Sex													
M													
F								×		×			
Geri	×												
Paed													
Acute						×							
Gene													
Derm													
Rheum							×						
Resp													×
Neuro					×								
Endo		×											
Eye					×				×				
ENT				×									
GI										×			
CVD			×			×							

Case	Description
1	Male carer; male partner ?dementia
2	Thyroid disease
3	Learning disabilities and heart failure
4	Tinnitus
5	Visual problems in bus driver; ?MS
6	Chest pain; ?MI, home visit
7	Shoulder pain
8	PV discharge; interpreter
9	Wants sick note; angry
10	Dyspepsia; offensive language
11	HRT; expert patient
12	Drug misuse
13	Lung cancer; breaking bad news

Examination 2 – Primary nature of each case

Station	Gender mix	Age mix	Skills in diagnosis	Ongoing management skills	Clinical practical skills	Health promotion	Diversity and ethical issues	Dealing with patients' emotions
1 Dementia – carer	M carer (absent patient)	72 – carer (68 – pt)					X	
2 Hypothyroidism	F	42	X					
3 Learning disabilities	F (absent patient)	50 – sister (44 – pt)					X	
4 Tinnitus	F	58			X			
5 ?MS	M	32	X					
6 Chest pain – home visit	M	74	X					
7 Shoulder pain	M	58			X			
8 PV discharge – using interpreter	F	38					X	
9 Wants sick note	M	58						X
10 Dyspepsia	F	38		X				
11 HRT	F	48		X				
12 Drug misuse	M	20				X		
13 Lung cancer; breaking bad news	M	72						X

Index

ACE inhibitors 80
acne 32–40
acromioclavicular joint disease 190
acupuncture, frozen shoulder 189
acute otitis media 59
adhesive capsulitis 182–91
adolescents 92–101
advance decisions, withholding health
   care 153
aggressiveness
  dementia 134
  see also angry patients
AIDS *see* HIV infection
alcohol 107, 108
  drug misuse and 232
Alzheimer's disease 128–36
amlodipine 78
amoxicillin, otitis media 59
analgesics, lower back pain 124
angina, fitness to drive 171
angiotensin converting enzyme
   inhibitors (ACE inhibitors) 80
angry patients 200–7
ankylosing spondylitis 125
antibiotics
  acne 39
  contraceptives and 34–5
  inappropriate use 52–60
antidepressants 8, 9
  menopausal symptoms 225
antihypertensive drugs 79
Applied Knowledge Test viii
arrhythmias, fitness to drive 171
aspirin
  hypertension 78, 79
  myocardial infarction 180
asthma 12–20
  fitness to drive 172
autoimmune hypothyroidism 145
autonomy of patients
  learning difficulties 148–55
  myocardial infarction 174–81
  teenagers 92–101
azelaic acid 39

back pain 118–26
bad news, breaking 238–45
bag, doctor's x
benzoyl peroxide 39
biceps tendon 188
Black patients 80

body image 37
body mass index (BMI) 29
brain tumours, fear of 156–63
breaking bad news 238–45
breast cancer, HRT risk 223, 225
British Medical Association, *Good
   Medical Practice for General
   Practitioners 2002* 69
British National Party 211
bronchial carcinoma 238–45
business commitments, self-care and
   110–16

calcium channel blockers 78, 80
cancer
  breaking bad news 238–45
  breast, risk from HRT 223, 225
  see also brain tumours, fear of
cannabis 232
capsulitis, adhesive 182–91
cardiovascular disease
  erectile dysfunction 49
  examination 87
  fitness to drive 171
  risk prediction charts 72–81
  valve disease 148–55
  see also coronary heart disease;
    hypertension; myocardial
    infarction
carers, support of 133–4
cauda equina syndrome 123
chest pain 174–81
cholesteatoma 57
cholesterol, cardiovascular disease risk
   77
chronic disease management 17, 20
chronic obstructive pulmonary disease
  fitness to drive 172
  smoking 238–45
'chunk and check' 186
  breaking bad news 242
  telephone consultations 114
clinical management skills xi
Clinical Skills Assessment viii–xv
clonidine 225
closed questions xiv
co-cyprindiol 38, 39
cognitive behavioural therapy,
   depression 9
colleagues, concerns about 62–71
colon, Crohn disease 110–16

combined oral contraceptives, acne and 38
communication skills 186
  breaking bad news 238–45
  explaining risk levels 223
  health beliefs and 77
  using interpreters 192–9
  see also telephone
competence limits (physician), drug misuse 233–4
complaints, about colleagues 62–71
complex cases 82–91
condoms 98
confidentiality, children 98–9
conjunctival haemorrhage 200–7
consent
  children 98–9
  learning difficulties and 153
consultations, simulated ix–x
contact *see* touch
contraceptives
  acne 38
  doxycycline 35, 37
  after menopause 224
  teenagers 98, 99
coronary heart disease
  HRT and 225
  see also myocardial infarction
corticosteroids *see* steroids
counselling, psychosexual 48
Crisis Mental Health Teams 8
Crohn's disease 110–16

'dangerous' diagnoses 180
data gathering skills xi
deafness 138–46
deep vein thrombosis (DVT), risk from HRT 225
delayed prescribing, antibiotics 59
demanding patients 52–60
dementia 128–36
  fitness to drive 172
denial mechanism 168
Department for Work and Pensions, sick notes 206
depression 2–10
diabetes mellitus 70
  fitness to drive 172
  frozen shoulder 189
diagnostic overshadowing 154
diamorphine (heroin)
  misuse 228–36
  myocardial infarction 180
Dianette (co-cyprindiol) 38, 39
Disability Discrimination Act 1995, hearing impairment 142

discriminatory language 208–16
dismissive patients 164–73
diversity issues 128–36, 208–16
  hearing impairment 138–46
dizziness 82–91
doctor's bag x
Down's syndrome 148–55
doxycycline, contraceptives and 35, 37
driving 170–1
  frozen shoulder 182–91
  hypertension 79
drugs
  misuse 228–36
  see also medications
DS 1500 (benefit form when potentially terminal illness) 207
DVLA 170–1
  hypertension 79

e-portfolios viii
ear
  pain 56–9
  see also hearing
elderly patients
  dizziness 82–91
  hypertension 79
emergencies
  back pain 123
  consent of children 99
  Crohn's disease 110–16
  myocardial infarction 174–81
emotional responses
  bad news 242
  negative 56, 204
employers, sick notes and 205
endocrine diseases, erectile dysfunction secondary to 49
endoscopy, indications in dyspepsia 215
epilepsy, fitness to drive 170
equality and diversity issues *see* diversity issues
equipment (doctor's bag) x
erectile dysfunction 42–51
erythromycin, otitis media 59
ethics
  advance decisions on withholding health care 153
  fitness to practise 62–71
  see also consent; diversity issues
ethnic minorities
  Black patients 80
  cardiovascular disease risk 77
  interpreters for 192–9
examinations (physical) *see* physical examinations
exercise, obesity and 27

expert patients 218–27
eye
 conjunctival haemorrhage 200–7
 thyroid disease 143
 vision, fitness to drive 170

family history
 breast cancer risk 223
 cardiovascular disease risk 77
Family Law Reform Act 1969 99
fasting blood glucose 70
fear of brain tumour 156–63
fear of redundancy 202
fertility 102–9
 perimenopausal 224
fistula, rectovaginal 192–9
fitness to practise 62–71
forensic history 233
frameworks, for consultations xii–xiii
frontotemporal lobe dementia 135
frozen shoulder 182–91

gastrointestinal tract, bleeding 187
General Medical Council, *Good Medical Practice 2006* 69
Gillick-competence 99
glandular fever 97
glenohumeral joint disease 190
glucose
 blood levels 70
 tolerance test 70
glue ear 59
glycaemia, impaired fasting 70
goitre 143
Good Medical Practice 2006 (General Medical Council) 69
grids, test frameworks xii–xiii, 247–50

H$_2$-receptor antagonists, endoscopy and 215
Hallpike test 87
Hashimoto's thyroiditis 145
health promotion
 fertility and 102–9
 obesity and 22–30
 young people 98
 see also lifestyle advice
healthcare teams, relationship breakdown 67–8
hearing
 assessment 57
 impairment 138–46
heart failure 148–55
heartburn 208–16
Helicobacter pylori, testing 214
hepatitis, vaccination 234

herbal remedies
 depression 8
 HRT alternatives 223
heroin (diamorphine)
 misuse 228–36
 myocardial infarction 180
hidden agenda 32–40, 92–101, 156–63
high-density lipoproteins (HDL), cardiovascular disease risk 77
history-taking
 depression 7
 forensic history 233
 joint disease 187
 reticent patients 96–7
 sexual history 47
 telephone consultations 114–15
 third parties 26–7, 132–3
HIV infection 98
home visits 174–81
hormone replacement therapy 218–27
hypertension 72–81
 fitness to drive 171
 hormone replacement therapy and 223
hypothyroidism 138–46

impaired fasting glycaemia 70
impaired glucose tolerance 70
impotence 42–51
incapacity benefit 189
indigestion 208–16
 analgesics and 124
infertility 102–9
instability, shoulder 190
interpersonal skills xi
interpreters 192–9
ischaemic heart disease *see* coronary heart disease; myocardial infarction
isotretinoin (Roaccutane) 34, 37–8, 39

knowledge base xiv
knowledgeable patients 218–27

language, offensive 208–16
language lines (telephone) 198
Lasting Powers of Attorney 135
learning disabilities 148–55
 associated conditions 154
levothyroxine 145
Lewy body dementia 135
lifestyle advice
 fertility issues 108
 hypertension 78
 menopausal symptoms 224
 obesity and 22–30
 see also health promotion
long-acting β$_2$-agonists (LABA) 19

lung cancer 238–45

magnetic resonance imaging (MRI),
    patient experience of 170
management skills (clinical) xi
managing uncertainty 87–8
marking system xi
McDonald criteria, multiple sclerosis
    170
Med 3, 4, 5, 6 (sick notes) 206, 207
medications
    on acne 37
    causing dyspepsia 215
    see also non-steroidal anti-
        inflammatory drugs
    for erectile dysfunction 50
    erectile dysfunction from 49
    interactions, levothyroxine 145
memory difficulties see dementia
menopause, hormone replacement
    therapy 218–27
Mental Capacity Act 2005 135
metoclopramide, diamorphine with 180
minor illnesses, patient education 58,
    60
mnemonics, chest pain 180
MRI (magnetic resonance imaging),
    patient experience of 170
multiple sclerosis 164–73
muscle relaxants, back pain 124
myocardial infarction 174–81
    fitness to drive 171

National Institute for Health and
    Clinical Excellence (NICE)
    guidelines
    depression 9
    hypertension 80
    obesity 29
neck, examination 143
negative emotional responses 56, 204
nerve root pain 125
neurological causes, erectile dysfunction
    49
non-steroidal anti-inflammatory drugs
    (NSAIDs)
    asthma 16
    indigestion 124, 187, 189
nurse practitioners 62–71
nurses, as patients 218–27

obesity, paediatrics 22–30
Objective Structured Clinical
    Examinations (OSCEs) ix
obstructive sleep apnoea, fitness to drive
    172

oestrogen-only HRT, risks 225
offensive language 208–16
open questions xiv
optic neuritis 164–73
osteoarthritis, back pain 125
otitis media 59
otoscopy 57
out-of-hours home visits 174–81
overshadowing, diagnostic 154
overweight, paediatrics 22–30

paediatrics 22–30
    teenagers 92–101
patient education, minor illnesses 58, 60
patient safety 67–8
patients, simulated xiv
peptic ulcer disease 187
perforation, tympanic membrane 57
performance assessment
    in workplace viii
    see also Clinical Skills Assessments
Personal Capability Assessment 206
phosphodiesterase type 5 inhibitors 50
physical activity, obesity and 27
physical examinations xi
    cardiovascular disease 87
    drug misuse 233
    shoulder 187–8
    spine 123–4
    thyroid disease 143
physiotherapy, frozen shoulder 189
Pick's disease 135
preparation for CSA viii–xv
proton pump inhibitors 189
    endoscopy and 215
psychogenic impotence 49
psychological effects, skin diseases 36
psychotic disorder, fitness to drive 172
pulmonary embolism, risk from HRT 225

racist language 208–16
random blood glucose 70
rectovaginal fistula 192–9
red flags
    back pain 123
    HRT complications 224
    shoulder 190
redundancy, fear of 202
referral requests 32–40
relatives 148–55
    see also third parties
relaxation techniques, hypertension 78
reticent patients 92–101
retinoids
    Roaccutane 34, 37–8, 39
    topical 38, 39

rheumatoid arthritis, back pain 125
Rinne's test 57–8
risk levels, explaining 223
Roaccutane (isotretinoin) 34, 37–8, 39
rotator cuff injury 188, 190
Royal College of General Practitioners,
    *Good Medical Practice for General
    Practitioners* 2002 69

safer sex 98
safety of patients 67–8
self-harm risk assessment 7
self-help 82–91
    tinnitus 161
sensate focused therapy 49
sensitive topics 46
sexual dysfunction 42–51
sexual history 47
sexual intercourse
    fertility 107, 108
    infection fear 92–101
sexual orientation 128–36
shoulder
    diagnosis flowchart 190
    frozen 182–91
sick doctors 62–71
sick notes 189, 200–7
    certificate types 206
simulated consultations ix–x
simulated patients xiv
simvastatin 78
skin diseases, psychological effects 36
sleep hygiene 161
smoking
    asthma 12–20
    cardiovascular disease risk prediction
        charts 76
    cessation 17–18, 107
    HRT and 223
    lung cancer 238–45
social effects, skin diseases 36
specialist drugs services 234
specialist referrals
    dyspepsia 215
    hypothyroidism 146
    requests from patients 32–40
spine 123–4, 125
St John's wort 8
statins 78, 79
stations, CSA ix–x
steroids
    inhaled 19
    joint injections 189

oral 18, 19
stroke, fitness to drive 170
substance misuse 228–36
suicide, risk assessment 7

talkative patients 118–26
tearful patients 2–10
teenagers 92–101
telephone
    consultations via 110–16
    language lines 198
terminal illness, definition 207
thiazides 78, 80
third parties 22–30, 128–36, 148–55
    see also relatives
thromboembolism, risk from HRT 225
thyroid disease 138–46
thyroxine (levothyroxine) 145
tibolone 225
timing, CSA procedure x
tinnitus 156–63
tiredness 138–46
total cholesterol, cardiovascular disease
    risk 77
touch 6
transient ischaemic attack, fitness to
    drive 170
translation services 192–9
triggers, asthma 16
trimethoprim, acne 39
tuning fork tests 57–8
tympanic membrane 57

uncertainty, managing of 87–8
urine samples, drug misuse 234

vaccination, injecting drug users 234
vaginal discharge 192–9
valve disease, cardiac 148–55
vascular dementia 135
venous thromboembolism, risk from
    HRT 225
vertebral collapse 125
vestibular sedatives 88
vision, fitness to drive 170

waist circumference 29
'warning shots', breaking bad news 242
Weber's test 58
workplace based assessment viii
'worried well' patients 109

yellow flags 123